Practical Radiography for Veterinary Nurses

Bicton College of Agriculture
26633   636. 0896 7572
Learning Resource Centre

Withdrawn   06/23

D1323805

WITHDRAWN

Commissioning editor: Mary Seager
Development editor: Caroline Savage
Production controller: Anthony Read
Desk editor: Jackie Holding
Cover designer: Fred Rose

Practical Radiography for Veterinary Nurses

Suzanne Easton

MSc Radiography (Imaging), BSC Radiography (Imaging)
Department of Clinical Veterinary Science, University of Bristol

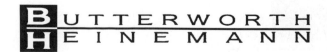

OXFORD AUCKLAND BOSTON JOHANNESBURG MELBOURNE NEW DELHI

Butterworth-Heinemann
Linacre House, Jordan Hill, Oxford OX2 8DP
225 Wildwood Avenue, Woburn, MA 01801-2041
A division of Reed Educational and Professional Publishing Ltd

ℛ A member of the Reed Elsevier plc group

First published 2002

Reed Educational and Professional Publishing Ltd 2002

All rights reserved. No part of this publication may be reproduced in
any material form (including photocopying or storing in any medium by
electronic means and whether or not transiently or incidentally to some
other use of this publication) without the written permission of the
copyright holder except in accordance with the provisions of the Copyright,
Designs and Patents Act 1988 or under the terms of a licence issued by the
Copyright Licensing Agency Ltd, 90 Tottenham Court Road, London,
England W1P 0LP. Applications for the copyright holder's written
permission to reproduce any part of this publication should be addressed
to the publishers

British Library Cataloguing in Publication Data
Easton, Suzanne
  Practical radiography for veterinary nurses
  1. Veterinary radiography
  I. Title
  636′.089′07572

ISBN 0 7506 5172 5

Typeset by Bath Typesetting, Bath
Printed and bound in Great Britain by MPG Books Ltd., Bodmin, Cornwall

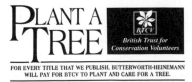

FOR EVERY TITLE THAT WE PUBLISH, BUTTERWORTH-HEINEMANN
WILL PAY FOR BTCV TO PLANT AND CARE FOR A TREE.

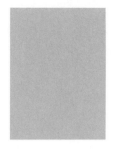

Contents

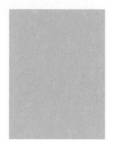

Acknowledgements

The completion of this book would not have been possible without the help and support of a number of people. I would firstly like to thank Dr Frances Barr for her encouragement and proof-reading throughout the progress of the book, from the initial proposal through to the finished draft. Also from the Department of Clinical Veterinary Science at the University of Bristol, I would like to thank Mr John Connibear and Mrs Tracey Dewey for their assistance in producing and digitizing all of the images used in the book and to Mrs Jeanne Latham for her support and as a source of valuable ideas.

I would also like to acknowledge the support provided by my husband, throughout the writing of this book, without whose culinary help the completion of the text would not have been possible.

Finally, I need to mention Kerry for her ongoing lap warming, Finn for his help with illegible typing and Teabag for his constant companionship.

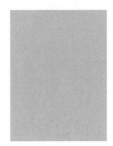

Foreword

It gives me great pleasure to write the foreword for this much-needed book on diagnostic radiography. Radiography is an integral part of veterinary practice today, whether dealing with small animals, horses, farm animals or exotic species. The images produced can provide invaluable diagnostic information, which can then be combined with facts gleaned from the history and the results of the physical examination and other diagnostic procedures to reach a definitive diagnosis. However, the potential yield of information depends on the production of a technically good image – and that is where this book will be so useful.

Maths and physics may have been forgotten or never clearly understood at school, but remain fundamental to understanding the principles of radiography. More specifically, it is vital to understand how the X-ray tube works, and how altering the exposure factors affects the X-ray beam produced. Only then can rational adjustments be made to the selected exposure factors to improve a sub-optimal image. Similarly, the steps involved in processing the X-ray film to produce a visible and permanent image must be clearly understood, so that imperfections in the process can be quickly detected and remedied.

Suzanne Easton trained as a radiographer in the human field, but has spent much of her working life to date working as a veterinary radiographer. She has been closely involved with teaching qualified veterinary nurses who are working towards the Diploma in Advanced Veterinary Nursing, and undergraduates aiming towards careers in veterinary nursing or veterinary surgery. She understands clearly, therefore, the theoretical and practical problems encountered by those studying radiography. The sections on radiographic techniques and radiation safety should enable all who read this book to work safely and effectively with X-rays. I commend it to you.

Frances Barr
MA VetMB PhD DVR DipECVDI MRCVS

Preface

Purpose

The purpose of this book is to provide a core of knowledge to assist in the understanding of radiography for veterinary nurses. The text provides information on the subjects covered in the veterinary nursing course and the advanced diploma in veterinary nursing. This is specific to the UK as there is no text currently available that focuses on positioning within the boundaries of the UK legislation or outlines and discusses the UK ionizing radiation legislation. This book also provides information useful to undergraduate veterinary surgeons, and will hopefully serve as a reference source for both qualified veterinary surgeons and nurses in practice.

Scope

The text deals with all aspects of radiography ranging from the basic principles of radiography and the mathematics involved, through to the principles of more sophisticated equipment and new techniques. It also covers the legislation for radiation protection and the impact this has on the veterinary practice. The manipulation of exposure factors and the production of a quality, diagnostic radiograph is discussed and includes film faults and imaging protocols as well as conventional positioning. Time is given to the care of equipment (processors, films, screens and the X-ray tube), that will hopefully be useful in the practice and will enhance the life of the equipment.

Approach

This book approaches radiography in a clear manner using a large number of line drawings and photographs. Key points are highlighted throughout and a set of revision points and questions is provided at the end of each chapter. The layout is easy to follow with each unit providing a 'stand-alone' section. It should be possible to use the book as a quick reference source of information as well as a textbook for initial learning and revision of radiography.

Essential mathematics and physics

Objectives

- Matter, energy, power and heat
- Units and prefixes used in radiography
- Radiological units
- Useful mathematics
- Proportions and the inverse square law

Introduction

This chapter will introduce and explore the principles of mathematics and physics that will make future chapters and principles of radiography easier to understand. Many of the concepts introduced in this chapter will be revision, but it is relevant to later chapters.

Matter, energy, power and heat

Matter

The entire world is made up of matter. Anything that occupies a space can be given this title. Matter is a collection of atoms and molecules, the basic building blocks. All matter has a mass, the measure of matter in an actual object. If gravity is involved, this mass is known as the weight of an object. If an object is placed outside of a gravitational field such as the atmosphere on the moon, the mass will remain the same, but the weight will decrease. The weight will also change if the object changes form, but again the mass will remain the same. An example of this is water in its three forms – solid (ice), liquid (water) and gas (steam). In these three forms the mass is the same throughout, but the weight changes considerably.

Matter	A collection of atoms and molecules
Mass	The measure of matter in an object
Weight	Mass under the influence of gravity

Energy

The process of matter altering state or form produces energy. Any object, however large or small, that is able to do work is said the have energy. Energy has a number of different forms (Table 1.1). Energy can be neither created nor destroyed although it can change from one form to another. Total energy is measured in joules (J).

Total energy = potential energy + kinetic energy

Table 1.1. Energy types, definitions and examples

Energy type	Description	Example
Potential	The amount of work an object could do because of its position	An axe raised, ready to be brought down to chop has potential energy
Kinetic	As an object leaves its state of potential energy it gains kinetic energy	An apple gains kinetic energy as it falls out of a tree
Electrical	The movement of electrons inside a conductor after the application of a potential difference	The movement of electrons in a cable produce the electrical energy needed to make a bulb light up
Nuclear	Nuclear energy is the energy stored within the nucleus of an atom	This energy is formed when the nucleus of an atom is split
Thermal	This is caused by the vibration of molecules within matter	A hot bath has faster moving molecules than a cool bath
Chemical	The energy generated when a reaction occurs between two substances	Thermal energy produced when water is added to hot oil
Electromagnetic	The interaction of electrons with matter, producing energy – the energy produced has specific characteristics*	X-ray production, radio waves, infrared light

*Characteristic radiation.

Power

Power is the rate of doing work or the rate of transforming energy. This is equivalent to joules per second or watts. In radiography, due to the amount of energy transformation occurring, power is measured in kilowatts.

Heat

Heat is the total energy of atoms and molecules moving in matter. The average speed of movement is known as temperature. Heat will always flow from hot to cold until equilibrium is reached. This movement can occur through three different methods – convection, conduction and radiation (Table 1.2). The rate of heat loss will depend on the type of surface material and the difference between the two areas of heat. This is utilized in an X-ray tube through the choice of material used for the anode and the colour of the tube head (black).

Table 1.2. Definitions of conduction, convection and radiation

Convection	This occurs in liquids and gasses. The matter moves taking the heat with it. This occurs due to the reduction in density associated with heating. Hotter material rises and displaces cooler material above. This is the principle behind surrounding an X-ray tube in oil as a cooling technique.
Conduction	This is found in metals. The heat is transferred through contact, with heat flowing from the hot area to the cooler area. This principle is used in the anode and stem of the X-ray tube.
Radiation	Vibrating molecules on the surface of matter generate electromagnetic waves. Energy in the form of heat leaves the surface and transfers the energy to whatever it strikes. This is most effective in a vacuum.

Units and prefixes used in radiography

The use of scientific terminology in radiography is based around standardized units and prefixes to abbreviate large or very small numbers and provides an international language between radiographers. The use of standardized units extends to the description of units of measure and the identification of units of ionizing radiation.

Standard scientific notation

Radiography uses both very large units and very small units. Examples of this are the 100 000 volts (V) necessary to radiograph a chest and the 0.004 amperes (A) needed to demonstrate a cat's carpus. These are two of the core units used in radiography and are described as kilovolts (kV) and milliamperes (mA). Using this notation, 100 000 V is described as 100 kV and 0.004 A as 4 mA. Where large numbers are used the numbers can also be described as exponents. Exponents describe numbers as multiples of 10 (the system most widely used in everyday life is the decimal system). The scientific notation relevant to radiography can be seen in Table 1.3.

Table 1.3. Standard scientific notation, prefixes and symbols

Notation	Decimal number	Prefix	Symbol
10^9	1 000 000 000	giga-	G
10^6	1 000 000	mega-	M
10^3	1000	kilo-	k
10^2	100	hecto-	h
10^1	10	deka-	da
10^{-1}	0.1	deci-	d
10^{-2}	0.01	centi-	c
10^{-3}	0.001	milli-	m
10^{-6}	0.000001	micro-	μ

SI base units

In order to maintain a common radiographic language the units used as a baseline for measurements and discussion need to be standardized.

Radiography uses the International System of Units or 'SI'. Problems would occur if the focus to film distance was given in metres on the practice exposure chart and the veterinary nurse carrying out examinations worked in inches. The base units in Table 1.4 are the units used to calculate more complicated measures such as speed ($m\,s^{-1}$) or force ($kg\,m\,s^{-2}$). There are seven base units from which all other units are derived.

Table 1.4. SI base units

Quantity	Name	Symbol
Mass	Kilogram	kg
Length	metre	m
Time	second	s
Electrical current	ampere	A
Temperature	kelvin	k
Luminous intensity	candela	cd
Amount of substance	mole	mol

Radiological units

Radiology has a number of units specific to the field that are in common use (Table 1.5). These are all related to the measurement of the production of X-rays, and the effect of the energy produced and used in diagnostic imaging. The units are mainly used in assessing and maintaining radiation safety or when discussing the use of the X-ray tube.

Table 1.5. Radiological units

Unit	Description	Symbol
kV_p	maximum energy of X-ray photons	kV_p
mA (mAs)	electron production in the X-ray tube	mA
KeV	kinetic energy of electrons in X-ray tube	keV
Heat unit	heat produced at anode kV_p mAs	HU
Gray	dose absorbed by a medium	Gy
Sievert	dose equivalent	Sv
Coulomb/kilogram	measure of atmospheric exposure	C/kg
Becquerel	radioactive disintegrations per second	Bq

kV_p

The potential difference between the cathode and anode in an X-ray tube is measured in kilovolts. This value determines the maximum energy of the X-ray photons emitted that will give the quality and intensity of the beam. In many machines this value may fluctuate and so the peak value is given (kV_p).

mA/mAs

In the production of X-rays, fast moving electrons must strike the anode within the X-ray tube. To produce these electrons, an electrical current must be applied to the cathode. This is measured in milliamperes. These electrons could be produced continuously, but this would cause damage to the tube and so the production of electrons is limited to a period of time (exposure time). The exposure time is expressed in mAs or milliamperes per second.

keV

As an electron is accelerated across the tube from the cathode to the anode it gains kinetic energy. This is measured in kiloelectron-volts. The keV will be the same as the kV_p.

Heat units

The production of X-rays produces heat at the anode. The amount of heat is specific to each exposure and can be calculated by multiplying the kV_p and mAs together. This is correct only if the voltage and current remain constant throughout the exposure.

Absorbed dose

The dose absorbed by the patient is measured as the gray (Gy). This is specific to the patient dose received and will vary according to the exposure used and the region being examined. The absorbed dose is the measurement of the energy absorbed by a medium.

Dose equivalent

The dose received by designated people working with radiation (dose equivalent) is measured in sieverts (Sv). This measurement is calculated by multiplying the grays received by a quality factor. The quality factor will take into account the different levels of damaged caused by radiation, and will alter depending on the type of ionizing radiations and the energy of the ionizing radiation. The dose equivalent is calculated from monitoring devices worn by personnel working with radiation.

Exposure in air

The amount of radiation in the atmosphere can be measured in coulomb/kilogram (C/kg). This measure of radiation can be only be used for air. The measure gives the total electric charge formed by ionization in one unit mass of air. This can be used for X-rays emerging from the tube or the intensity of gamma-rays during a scintigraphic examination.

Activity

The final radiographic unit is the becquerel (Bq). Radioactive substances have unstable nuclei and try to change the structure of the nucleus to a more stable structure. Each change in structure is called disintegration. The becquerel measures the number of changes per second.

Useful mathematics

Day to day radiography involves mathematics. This may be simple addition or multiplication, but can also involve fractions and ratios. As a simple 'aide memoire', this section will demonstrate the basic mathematics essential to radiography in Table 1.6, where a and b denote any number, and x is any number that you wish to calculate.

Table 1.6. Useful mathematics

Description	How to do it
Percentage change	$100\ (b - a/a)$
Percentage of b compared to a	$100\ b/a$
x as a percentage of a	$(x/100)\ a$
Parts of a fraction	Numerator $\quad a$ denominator $\quad b$
Adding and subtracting fractions	Find a common denominator and then add or subtract the numerators
Multiplying fractions	Multiply numerators and denominators
Dividing fractions	Turn the second fraction upside down and then multiply
Ratios	Demonstrates the relationship between two related measures, e.g. kV : X-rays produced
Decimals	A fraction that has a denominator that can be divided by 10 can be shown as a decimal, e.g. $5/10 = 0.5$
To calculate x when a and b are known, divide both known numbers by the multiple of x When a known number is added to x, subtract the known number from both sides When x is part of a fraction, cross multiply	$ax = b$ $ax/a = b/a$ $x = b/a$ $x + a = b$ $x + a - a = b - a$ $x = b - a$ $x/a = b/c$ $xc = ab$ $x = ab/c$
Cross multiplication	

Proportions and the inverse square law

Proportions

Measurements can be either directly or indirectly proportional. If two measurements are directly proportional, the ratio of one to the other is constant.

$a/b = $ constant

If something is described as being inversely proportional, the factors will be inverted. As one factor increases the other will decrease or *vice versa*.

$a \times b = \text{constant}$

Inverse square law

The intensity of radiation from a given point is inversely proportional to the square of the distance between that point and the source. This means that the greater the distance between the two points, the weaker the intensity. This plays an important role in radiation safety. The greater the distance between yourself and the source of radiation, the lower the dose you will receive.

$I\alpha\ 1/d^2$

The effect distance has on the exposure is determined by the inverse square law. As the distance of the object from the source increases, the intensity of the radiation will decrease. If you double the distance, the exposure intensity decreases by a factor of 4. This can be seen in a similar way using a torch beam. The closer the wall is to the torch beam, the stronger the intensity of the beam against the wall. As you move away from the wall, the beam will be weaker when it hits the wall (see Figure 1.1).

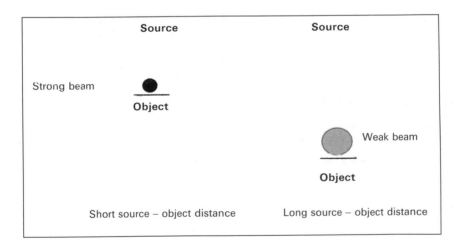

Figure 1.1. The inverse square law demonstrated using a torch beam against a wall.

Revision questions

1. How are mass and matter related?
2. What is weight?
3. List and give examples of three types of energy
4. What is 30,000 volts in kilovolts?
5. What is 4.5 mA in decimal notation?
6. What name is given to the unit of measure for time?
7. Give the measure of absorbed dose and describe what the measurement demonstrates
8. Describe the calculation of a becquerel
9. What is the symbol for a Sievert?
10. What is a ratio?
11. Add 4/5 to 3/7
12. Divide 3/10 by 1/8
13. Work out the following equations $x + 10 = 37$

$$4x = 24$$
$$x/8 = 3/4$$

14. If a is inversely proportional to b, what will happen to a if b doubles?
15. Using the inverse square law and thinking about an X-ray beam, if you double your object source distance what will have happened to the intensity and size of the beam when it reaches the object?

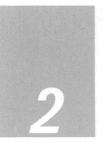

The principles of physics used in radiography

2

Objectives

- Electrostatics – the electric charge
- Conductors and insulators
- Electricity
- Measuring electricity
- Types of current
- Laws of an electric current
- Resistance
- Making a circuit – the options
- Magnetism
- The function and composition of a magnet
- Magnetic laws
- Electromagnetism – electricity and magnetism in union
- Laws of electromagnetic induction

Introduction

Although the essential use of electricity is immediately obvious in radiography, i.e. the conversion of electric energy into electromagnetic energy, it also has a subtle role, not always considered immediately. Electricity and magnetism are both utilized in the stages leading up to the current and potential difference being available for use in the correct form within the X-ray tube. If the two concepts are not understood and related back to the processes involved in the production of X-rays, an understanding of technical and practical procedures will not be possible.

Electrostatics – the electric charge

This imposing term is used to describe the study of electrical charges. These charges are all around and experienced daily. These static electrical charges are seen in many forms – as discharges during storms as lightning through to uncontrollable hair after it has been washed! (see Figure 2.1).

An electric charge is created when a negatively charged electron is removed from a positive proton in the nucleus of an atom. The electron removed is a

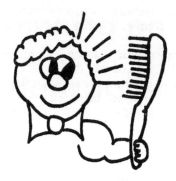

Figure 2.1. The effects of static on washed hair!

free electron that is very loosely bound to the atom and easy to remove. The simplest way to remove these free electrons is through friction. Other methods of electron removal include heat, which is the method used in the X-ray tube, and induction, the use of the electrical field of a charged object to transfer charge to an uncharged object. Charges are of two types – positive or negative. The electron will always be negatively charged and the proton always positively charged. The electron and proton are the smallest units of charge. They will have equal magnitude, but opposite signs.

The force between two charges can be calculated using the inverse square law. As the distance between the two charges increases, the force will decrease. However, this will depend on the medium the atom is suspended in and is not constant. Force will be present even when a vacuum separates the atoms.

Charge is measured in coulombs (Q). One coulomb is equivalent to 6×10^{18} electrons. This is also known as the electromotive force.

Free electrons	Loosely bound electrons in an atom
Positive charge	Created by a proton being separated from an electron
Negative charge	Created by removing an electron from a proton
Force	Between charges forces will always be equal and opposite
Coulomb	Measure of charge 1 Coulomb = 6×10^{18} electrons

Conductors and insulators

Materials are either conductors or insulators. If the material has free electrons, then it is a conductor. This is usually a material composed of metallic elements. A conductor can be charged through heating, friction or induction. If a conductor is placed in an electrical circuit, then charge will flow through the circuit including the conductor. Examples of conductors include metals such as copper, titanium and aluminium, the earth, and the human body.

If a material has very few free electrons, then it will be an insulator. In an insulator, any charge produced on the surface will not move along the material. The charge will remain where it is formed. If the material is placed into a circuit, then no charge will be present, as the material will not allow electrons to flow. Examples of insulators include plastics, rubber, glass and silicon.

Insulators	Very few free electrons
Conductors	Free electrons present allowing easy release and movement of electrons

Electricity

A potential difference must occur to achieve current flow. If a piece of wire is joined between a positive and negative point, a potential difference is formed. If a potential difference is present across a piece of wire, then weakly bound electrons will flow through the wire. This is an electrical current.

Measuring electricity

Electricity is measured in volts. This is the potential difference within the circuit, which must be present if a current is to flow.

Volts = joules/coulomb

Two points within a circuit have a potential difference of 1 V if 1 J of work is done for every coulomb of electricity passing between the two points.

Every part of a circuit has a maximum potential difference that it is able to produce. This is called the electromotive force. This is measured in volts in the same way as potential difference.

The power of electricity is measured in watts (W). One watt is equal to 1 A of current flowing through an electric potential of 1 V. Household appliances usually need about 500–1000 W to work effectively. An X-ray machine usually needs 30–100 kW of power to work efficiently.

Watts = Amperes × voltage

Types of current

Current takes two forms, either alternating or direct. In a circuit with a direct current, the electrons flow in one direction only. This provides a continuous flow that is demonstrated with a straight waveform on a graph (Figure 2.2). The distance between the time axis and the horizontal line of the current will determine the magnitude of the current.

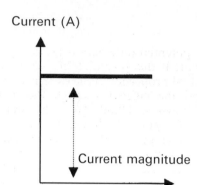

Figure 2.2. Waveform generated by a direct current.

Alternating current will produce a sinusoidal waveform, with the flow of the current fluctuating between two directions (Figure 2.3). The electrons first move in one direction to their maximum 'positive' potential and then in the reverse direction back to the opposite maximum 'negative' potential.

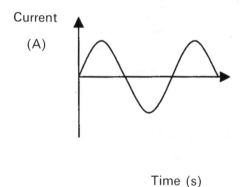

Figure 2.3. Waveform generated by an alternating current.

Laws of an electric current

- An electrical potential difference must be present
- There must be a complete circuit around which the electrons can flow
- Current will always flow from positive to negative (whilst electron flow is always from negative to positive)

Resistance

As is already known, a potential difference is necessary to allow current to pass through a conductor. If this potential difference increases the current increases. If all the physical properties of the conductor remain constant the potential difference and the current through the material will remain proportional. This is known as Ohm's law. The units of resistance are measured in ohms (Ω). If a graph is drawn demonstrating resistance, the gradient will be constant (Figure 2.4). If the physical properties of the conductor are altered, e.g. temperature changes in a light bulb, the gradient of the graph will alter (Figure 2.5). The resistance through a wire can also be altered if the thickness of the wire is altered. Therefore, the thinner the wire, the greater the resistance.

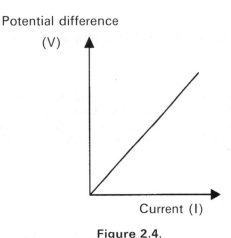

Figure 2.4.

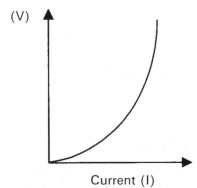

Figure 2.5.

Making a circuit – the options

When a circuit is designed a number of different components can be added to alter the function of the circuit of the flow of charge through the circuit. The combinations are extensive, but the key elements used in radiography are outlined in Table 2.1.

Table 2.1. Components of electrical circuits

Circuit component	Function	Symbol
Battery	provides a source of electrical potential	
Ammeter	measures electrical current	
Voltmeter	measures electrical potential	
Switch	turns a circuit on or off by providing a means for the electrons to flow in a complete circuit	
Resistor	slows or reduces the flow of electrons	
Rheostat	a resistor that can have the amount of flow it will allow altered	
Diode	this will restrict the flow of electrons to one direction only	
Transformer	if the current is alternating the voltage will be increased or decreased by a certain amount	
Capacitor	this is able to store electrical charge; used in some portable X-ray machines	

Magnetism

Magnetic materials are found naturally in nature. The name originates from the discovery of magnetic iron oxide in the village of Magnesia in Western Turkey. More recently alloys have been manufactured that can be made into very strong magnets.

Magnetism   The ability of certain materials to attract iron

The function and composition of a magnet

Every magnet has a pole. This is where the lines of force are most concentrated. An area called the magnetic field surrounds the poles (Figure 2.6). Poles will always be found in pairs.

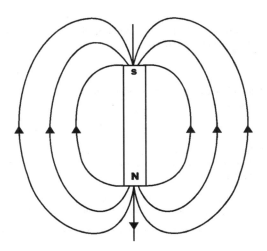

Figure 2.6. Magnetic lines of force due to north and south poles.

In a magnetic field force can be exerted on another pole. The simplest example of these forces is seen in a bar magnet (Figure 2.7).

Figure 2.7. Magnetic fields around a bar magnet.

Any charged particle that is moving will have a magnetic field. If the movement of the electron is contained in the nucleus of an atom, the lines of the magnetic field will be perpendicular to the movement of the electron. Electrons will circle the nucleus in either a clockwise or anticlockwise direction. This is known as electron spin. If the wire is circular, the fields will flow in a similar way to those in a bar magnet.

Types of magnets

Magnets fall into two categories – temporary and permanent. A permanent magnet retains its magnetism. The north pole is always the same and will attract other permanent magnets and other magnetic materials.

A temporary magnet looses its magnetism by movement or heating. In some temporary magnets, the force needed to loose magnetism is very small.

Ferromagnetism

Ferromagnetism is the most commonly encountered magnetism in radiography. It is found in transformers and electromagnetic relays. Ferromagnets are found in large quantities in substances such as iron, nickel and cobalt. In these materials the atoms are arranged into 'magnetic domains'. Within each domain the atoms are all pointing in the same direction, although all the domains may not be in a similar direction.

An electromagnet is composed of several coils of copper wire around a soft iron core. This coil is called a solenoid. A current is then applied to the wire and an electromagnet is formed.

Magnetic laws

Magnets have a number of laws that are similar to electrostatics and gravity, but are specific to magnets alone.

Attraction and repulsion

The lines of magnetic field will always exit the magnet from the north pole and flow to the south pole. When placed within the magnetic field of another magnet, like poles will repel and opposing poles will attract.

Existence of poles in pairs

As is the case on the earth, there will always be two poles. If a magnet is cut or broken in half, two new, smaller magnets will be made, still with two poles (Figure 2.8).

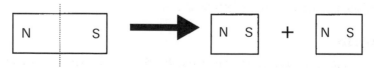

Figure 2.8. The effect of cutting a bar magnet in half.

Magnetic induction

A material that can be easily magnetized, ferromagnetic material, is made up of lots of individual small magnets called dipoles. The dipoles are scattered randomly through the material. If a ferromagnetic material is placed in a magnetic field, the dipoles will arrange themselves in line with the flow of the magnetic field (Figure 2.9).

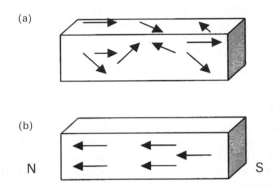

Figure 2.9. Effect of a magnet on the dipoles of ferromagnetic material. (a) Ferromagnetic material with randomly orientated magnetic dipoles. (b) Ferromagentic material under the influence of a magnet.

Magnetic flux

Magnetic flux is the number of lines of magnetic force passing through a given area. This will vary depending on the density of the material it is passing through. This is described in teslas (T). This is important in the classification of magnetic resonance imaging (MRI) scanners.

Electromagnetism – electricity and magnetism in union

Electromagnetism is the production of electricity by a changing magnetic field. The most basic example of this is the production of electricity using a dynamo. The placing of a conductor into a magnetic field will produce an electromotive force in that conductor. The greater the strength of magnetic field and the speed of the introduction and removal of the conductor from the magnetic field will alter the size of electromotive force generated.

Laws of electromagnetic induction

There are two laws directly related to electromagnetic induction. These can be calculated using Fleming's left-hand rule.

Faraday's law

Whenever the is a change in the magnetic flux linked with a circuit and electromotive force is induced, the strength of which is proportional to the rate of change of the flux through the circuit.

Lenz's law

The direction of the induced current is always such as to oppose the change producing it.

Fleming's left-hand rule

Magnetic fields around currents will have an individual anticlockwise magnetic field around every electron. The direction of the magnetic field in relation to the electron flow can be demonstrated using Fleming's left-hand rule (Figure 2.10).

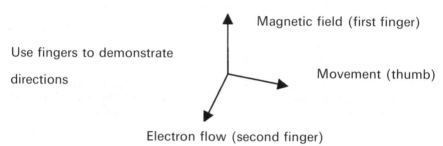

Use fingers to demonstrate

directions

Magnetic field (first finger)

Movement (thumb)

Electron flow (second finger)

Figure 2.10. Fleming's left hand rule.

Revision points
- Electric charge – current time
- An object becomes charged by the addition or removal of electrons – this can be caused by friction, contact or induction.
- Laws of electricity:
  - Unlike charges attract, like charges repel.
  - When an object become charged the charges are spread evenly throughout the object
- Potential energy of electricity is measured in the Volt (V)
- Conductors – allow easy flow of electrons
- Insulators – assist the flow of electrons
- Currents and circuits – Electrons flow on the outer surface of a wire. If the wire is in contact at both ends an electrical circuit is made. The number of electrons flowing in this circuit is measured in amperes (A)
- Direct current – electrons flow in one direction along the conductor
- Alternating current – electrons flow in one direction and then the other
- Magnetism – A charged moving particle creates a magnetic field. The electrons around the nucleus can be orientated in the same direction using a magnet. Magnetic force will always flow from south to north
- Magnetic laws:
  - Opposites attract
  - Non-magnetic materials can be made magnetic through induction (bringing it into the field around a magnetic material
  - Every magnet, however small, will have two poles
- Electromagnetic induction – the production of electricity in a magnetic field

Review questions

1. *How can an electric charge be produced? Give two ways.*
2. *What is the simplest way to release free electrons?*
3. *What unit is charge described in?*
4. *Conductors are mainly what type of material?*
5. *Name two everyday insulators.*
6. *What must be present to allow a current to flow?*
7. *What unit is potential difference measured in?*
8. *Draw a graph to demonstrate the current flow in an alternating current*
1. *What is resistance measured in?*
10. *Does a thin wire have high or low resistance when compared to a thick wire?*
11. *Draw the symbol for the part of an electric circuit that will only allow current to flow in one direction*
12. *If two similar poles of two magnets are brought into close proximity what will happen?*
13. *Name the material that could be used for the core of an electromagnet*
14. *If a conductor is brought in and out of a magnetic field, what happens?*
15. *Name the two laws relating to electromagnetic induction.*

3 Inside the atom

Objectives

- Atoms, elements and other definitions
- The 'make-up' of an atom
- Shells and energy
- The periodic table
- Radioactivity
- The effects of an electron changing orbits
- Photons and their movement
- Frequency and wavelength
- The electromagnetic spectrum
- Properties of ionizing radiation

Introduction

The concepts and ideas discussed in this chapter can prove daunting at first. If the concepts are thought of as a miniature solar system, something that can actually be visualized, then the theory will become more manageable and less of a difficulty. The topics in this chapter cannot be shown with photographs or actual props, and so a good imagination and acceptance of the work of others is essential.

Atoms will join the theory of matter with ionizing radiation, to form the base of radiography built in previous chapters to be taken into future chapters.

Atoms, elements and other definitions

See Table 3.1.

The 'make-up' of an atom

The atom is the basic unit involved in the production and use of X-rays. Unless a vacuum has been created, atoms are present in every solid, liquid and gas.

Jo Coleman

Information Update Service

Butterworth-Heinemann

FREEPOST SCE 5435

Oxford

Oxon

OX2 8BR

UK

FOR CARDS
OUTSIDE
THE UK.
PLEASE
AFFIX A
POSTAGE STAMP

Keep up-to-date with the latest books in your field.

Visit our website and register now for our **FREE** e-mail update service, or join our mailing list and enter our monthly prize draw to win £100 worth of books. Just complete the form below and return it to us now! (FREEPOST if you are based in the UK)

www.bh.com

Please Complete In Block Capitals

Title of book you have purchased:...

....

Subject area of interest:...

Name:..

Job title:...

Business sector (if relevant):...

Street:...

Town:.. County:...

Country:.. Postcode:..

Email:...

Telephone:..

How would you prefer to be contacted: Post ☐   e-mail ☐   Both ☐

Signature:... Date:...

☐ Please arrange for me to be kept informed of other books and information services on this and related subjects (✔ box if not required). This information is being collected on behalf of Reed Elsevier plc group and may be used to supply information about products by companies within the group.

FOR OFFICE USE ONLY

Butterworth-Heinemann,
a division of Reed Educational
& Professional Publishing Limited.
Registered office: 25 Victoria Street,
London SW1H 0EX.
Registered in England 3099304.
VAT number GB: 663 3472 30.

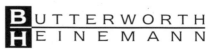

A member of the Reed Elsevier plc group

Table 3.1. Terms relating to atoms

Term	Symbol	Definition
Atom		The smallest unit of an element that has the specific properties of the element
Atomic number	Z	The number of protons in a nucleus
Atomic mass number	A	The total number of protons or neutrons in the nucleus of an atom
Neutron number	N	The number of neutrons within the nucleus
Element	E	A nucleus with a set, known atomic number
Molecule		Atoms from different elements combined – molecules can be seen in the form of water, H_2O [two hydrogen atoms (H) and an oxygen atom (O) combined] or salt, NaCl [one sodium atom (Na) and one chlorine atom (Cl) combined]
Compound		The substance formed when two or more molecules join together
Isotope		An atom with the same atomic number, but a different atomic mass number and number of neutrons as a given element
Isobar		An atom with the same atomic mass number as a given element, but a different atomic number and number of neutrons in the nucleus
Radioisotope		A nucleus of an atom with particular atomic mass and atomic mass number that is radioactive

The atomic nucleus

Atoms are composed of a nucleus that contains protons and neutrons. Protons are positively charged. Neutrons have no electrical charge. Electrons surround the nucleus of an atom (see Figure 3.1).

Protons and neutrons are about 2000 times bigger than electrons. For this reason the mass of an atom is almost completely made up of the protons and

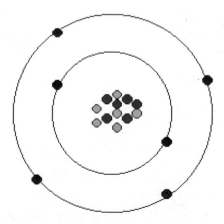

Figure 3.1. The structure of a carbon atom.

neutrons in its nucleus. The total number of protons and neutrons in the nucleus is known as the mass number. Forces known as short-range forces hold the nucleus together. These are very strong forces. The energy used in keeping the nucleus together is called a binding energy.

Shells and energy

The electrons orbit around the nucleus in different planes; these planes are called shells. The shells nearest the nucleus will always be the first to be completely full. This is because they have lower energy levels and are easier to fill. If there are not enough electrons to fill the shell, then the odd electrons will be found in the outermost shell. Each shell has a maximum number of electrons that it can hold, before the next shell is entered. If the outer shell is full, the atom will be stable. If the shell is not full, the atom will attempt to gain electrons to fill the outer shell. This will make the atom unstable (see Table 3.2).

Table 3.2. Numbers of electrons in atomic shells

Shell number	Shell Letter	Maximum number of electrons
1	K	2
2	L	8
3	M	18
4	N	32

The periodic table

All elements known to man are arranged in the periodic table. This table displays all the elements in groups according to their chemical and physical properties. Group I is composed of the alkali metals (excluding hydrogen), which combine easily with oxygen and react violently with water. Elements in Group VIII are called the noble gases. These do not react with other elements easily. By convention, the periodic table will show the atomic mass and atomic number of every element. The atomic number will always be above the symbol for the element and the mass number will always be below the element symbol. Using the periodic table, the number of electrons, protons and neutrons in an atom can be calculated (Figure 3.2).

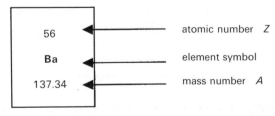

Figure 3.2. Single unit from the periodic table (barium).

Radioactivity

Any nucleus that is unstable is said to be radioactive. The nucleus will attempt to change the internal structure to a more stable form resulting sometimes in the ejection of a charged particle from the nucleus. Every time the nucleus changes its structure it is called a radioactive disintegration or transformation. This may result in a change to the atomic number, the atomic mass number or both. If the atomic number is changed, then the resulting element will be different. It is not possible to predict which atom in a sample will change its internal structure – the disintegration of an atom is a random event.

Elements with a high mass number are more likely to consist of isotopes and therefore undergo a change in nucleus structure. This is because these elements have atoms with far more neutrons than protons. This excess in neutrons will lead to instability.

The effects of an electron changing orbits

Although electrons are usually found in the orbits surrounding the nucleus with the innermost shells filled, this is not always the case. An electron within an atom can undergo a collision or interaction at any time. This event will alter the energy level of the electron producing either excitation or ionization. The unit of electromagnetic radiation produced during this interaction is known as a photon or quantum.

Excitation

Interactions can occur that will give the electron enough energy to move from one orbit to an outer orbit. This is known as excitation. This 'excited' electron is then able to return to its original orbit, releasing a photon of electromagnetic radiation as it goes (Figure 3.3).

Ionization

Ionization occurs when an electron is subjected to enough energy to remove

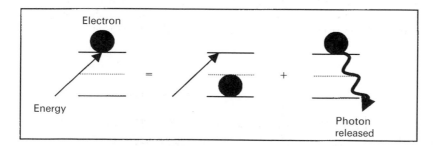

Figure 3.3. The excitation of an electron and the release of a photon of electromagnetic radiation.

it from the atom completely. The electron is 'free' and has a kinetic energy (Figure 3.4). The ejected electron and the positive atom are called an ion pair.

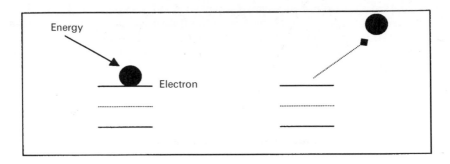

Figure 3.4. The effects of ionization on the position of an electron in an atom.

Characteristic radiation

Characteristic radiation is the excess energy formed and given off or emitted when an electron moves into a different shell to make the new shell complete. This is a discrete package of energy in the form of radiation and is measured in quanta of energy photons (keV). This energy level will not remain constant.

Frequency and wavelength

Wavelength and frequency relates to any form of wave. In the context of radiography this is the electromagnetic spectrum.

Wavelength (λ)

A wavelength is the distance between two consecutive peaks or troughs during the movement of a wave of any type.

Frequency (ν)

Frequency is the number of cycles of the wave passing a fixed point per second and is measured in Hertz (Hz). This is inversely proportional to the wavelength.

The smaller the wavelength, the higher the frequency or energy of the wave (Figure 3.5).

As frequency and wavelength are inversely proportional, an increase in wavelength will result in a decrease in frequency. To remember these changes think of trying to run taking large strides and how it is not possible. Your stride size relates to the wavelength and your speed of movement the frequency.

1 Wavelength (λ)

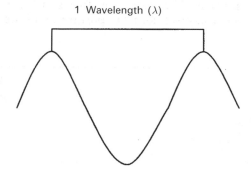

Figure 3.5. Electromagnetic wave.

The electromagnetic spectrum

The electromagnetic spectrum consists of waves of vibrations of electric and magnetic fields all with the same speed. This is the speed of light in a vacuum, which is 3×10^8 m s^{-1}. As it is always the same it is known as a constant (C). The difference between them is in their frequency and wavelength. The waves will always travel in straight lines, which is important for the inverse square law (see Table 3.3).

Table 3.3. The electromagnetic spectrum

Wavelength	Type	Production	Example
$> 10^{-4}$	Radio	Electrons oscillating in wires	Radio signal
7×10^{-7} to 10^{-4}	Infrared	Hot objects	Energy from the sun
4×10^{-7} to 7×10^{-7}	Visible	Very hot objects	
10^{-9} to 4×10^{-7}	Ultraviolet	Arcs and gas discharges	Light bulb
10^{-12} to 10^{-8}	X-rays	Electrons hitting metal target	
$< 10^{-10}$	y-rays	Radioactive nuclei	

A radio wave has a long wavelength and a low frequency
X-rays have a short wavelength and a high frequency
X-rays with a shorter wavelength will have more penetrating power than those with a long wavelength

Planck's constant

X-Ray photons will travel at the speed of light, and will either exist and have a velocity or will not exist at all. The energy of an X-ray photon is directly proportional to the frequency of the photon. This is Planck's constant (*h*).

$E \ (eV) = h \times f$
Photon energy (eV) = Planck's constant × photon frequency

Revision points

- Atom: Smallest unit within an element, but having all the properties. Made up of a nucleus containing neutrons and protons surrounded by electrons
- Molecules – combination of different atoms to make a structure, e.g. hydrogen and oxygen make water
- Compound – combination of different molecules
- Periodic table – table containing details of all elements known to man
- Shells and energy – Electrons orbit around the nucleus in shells. These hold a certain number of electrons per shell. If the shell is not complete the atom will react differently to an atom with a full outer shell
- Radioactivity – the emission of particles from an atom with an unstable nucleus with the aim of becoming stable (this emission is called radioactive decay)
- Ionization – The interaction of radiation with matter. This involves the removal of an electron from an atom. The ejected electron and the positive atom are called and ion pair
- Frequency – the rate of rise and fall of a wave (electromagnetic radiation travels in waves) is called the frequency – measured in hertz (Hz)
- Wavelength – the distance from crest to crest of the wave. If the frequency is high, the wavelength is short
- Electromagnetic spectrum – collection of radiation types with a range of frequencies – includes visible light, radio waves and X-rays

---

Revision questions

1. *What are the small discrete packets of electromagnetic radiation called?*
2. *What does the atomic number of an atom depend upon?*
3. *What is the term given to the positively charged particles contained within the nucleus of an atom?*
4. *What is a molecule?*
5. *How many electrons should there be in the innermost shell of an atom?*
6. *If an atom gains or loses one or more electrons, what it is called?*
7. *Name two parts of the electromagnetic spectrum*
8. *What does the nucleus of an atom contain?*
9. *If the frequency of a wavelength is high is it long or short?*
10. *What is the unit measure of frequency?*

4 The construction of an X-ray unit

Introduction

The equipment for the production of X-rays entails more than just the X-ray tube. A circuit is necessary to supply the electricity to allow the function of the X-ray tube. This chapter will concentrate on the parts that make up the rest of the X-ray 'machine'.

The X-ray circuit

The X-ray circuit is made up of a number of constituent parts. In isolation they perform no useful function, but when joined together the end result is the production of X-rays. The constituent parts may be compacted in a portable machine for easy use and mobility or may be found in separate rooms if the machine is fixed. The X-ray circuit should not be subjected to 'DIY' maintenance. The parts are delicate and easily damaged, and most importantly use very high voltages that may prove fatal if a qualified engineer does not carry out maintenance. A schematic diagram of the circuits involved in an X-ray machine is shown in Figure 4.1.

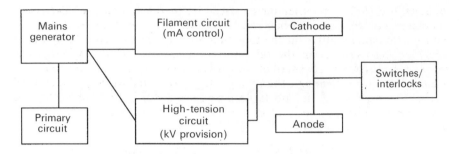

Figure 4.1. Schematic diagram of an X-ray machine.

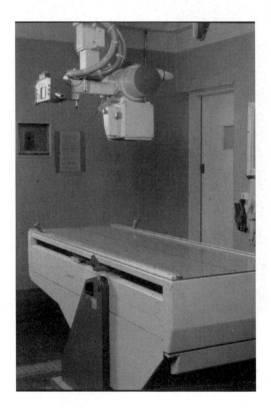

Figure 4.2. Fixed 'over-couch' X-ray machine.

What is seen from the outside?

From the outside the X-ray tube and the supporting circuits are very non-descript. If the machine is fixed, the generator will be visible as a large box off to one side of the room or under the table. These types of machines will also have a fixed consol from which the exposure factors can be set and the exposure actually made. These consoles will also have the mains voltage compensator and any other meters essential to the function of the X-ray machine. Portable and mobile machines will have the generator and the console contained either on the tube mounting or on the main body of the machine, separated from the tube by an extendable supporting arm. The X-ray tube itself is fairly small in comparison to the rest of the 'machine'. In mobile and fixed machines, the tube is usually rounded in shape, supported on a movable arm. In portable machines, the X-ray tube may be incorporated into the body of the 'machine', with no visible, specific tube region (see Figures 4.2–4.4).

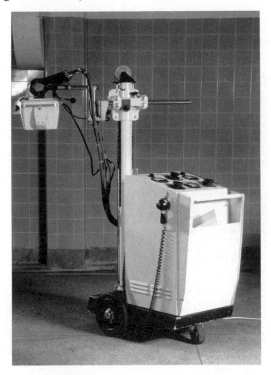

Figure 4.3. Mobile X-ray machine.

High-voltage generators

The generator is responsible for converting the mains voltage supply into a form that is suitable for use in the X-ray machine. In the X-ray tube, electrons cannot be accelerated from the anode to the cathode without causing major damage to the tube. For this reason the current entering the tube must flow in one direction only.

The electrical energy used in a generator comes from mechanical energy. This effect will produce a kV with a suitable waveform. The current supplied by the mains is alternating. This means that the average voltage is zero. To overcome this and provide a constant voltage from a constantly reversing current rectification is necessary.

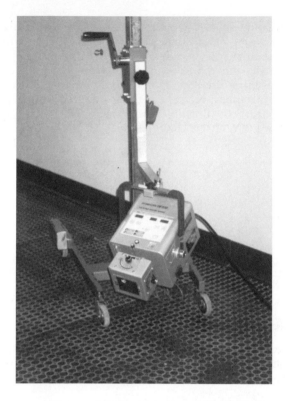

Figure 4.4. Portable X-ray machine.

Generator	Provides a constant voltage supply to the X-ray machine

Rectification

Rectification will provide a current that does alternate. The curve of a sine wave is known to fluctuate evenly between positive and negative during one cycle. If a rectifier is placed into the circuit, during the positive portion of the AC waveform, the rectifier will allow electrons to flow and pass through the X-ray tube. During the negative part of the waveform, the rectifier will not conduct and no current will flow. Rectification will occur through the use of a diode, a small electrical component that will allow flow of current in one direction only.

Half-wave rectification

Through the use of rectification, the negative half of the cycle can be eliminated. This is known as half-wave rectification. The main disadvantage of half-wave rectification is the loss of half the useful current. If the voltage passing through the rectifier is negative then no current will flow (see Figure 4.5).

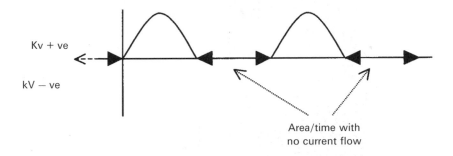

Figure 4.5. Half-wave rectification.

Full-wave rectification

If two separate pulses pass through a circuit for every cycle (one entire wavelength), the circuit is fully rectified. This will provide a positive voltage at all times across the X-ray tube (see Figure 4.6).

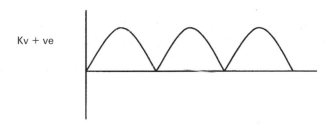

Figure 4.6. Full-wave rectification.

Three-phase power

All of the waveforms described above are produced by a single-phase power source that will produce a pulsating X-ray beam. To eliminate this effect, three simultaneous voltage waveforms can be produced out of step with one another. This will produce three-phase electric power. If this three-phase electric waveform is then rectified, a near constant high voltage is maintained. The voltage generated in this way never drops to zero (see Figure 4.7).

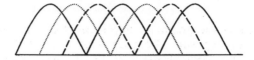

Figure 4.7. Three-phase waveforms with rectification.

High-frequency generator

The development of generators has led to the introduction of high-frequency generators. These generators have full-wave rectification and the frequency of the power is 500–25 000 Hz. The voltage waveform is almost constant. These generators are very small and can be placed within the X-ray tube housing. The resultant images have a better quality for a lower dose to the patient when compared to a conventional generator.

Half-wave rectification	Eliminates the negative phase of the current cycle
Full-wave rectification	The negative part of the cycle is inverted to give a positive voltage at all times
Three-phase power	Three simultaneous waveforms produced out of step
Three-phase rectification	Three-phase power, rectified to give a near constant voltage
High-frequency generators	Near constant waveform with a high frequency

Mains supply switch

This switch will isolate all equipment in an emergency and at the end of use. This switch contains a fuse (short piece of wire) that will melt if an abnormally high current flows through the fuse. The switch handle is connected to a copper rod with connectors. The connectors must make contact with the circuitry of the generator to allow a current to flow. The switch also has a spring to prevent accidental use.

Primary circuit

The primary circuit contains all of the meters necessary to determine the exposure being set prior to an exposure being made. These meters must not affect the reading while they measure the flow of electrons. The internal resistance of the circuit is kept to a minimum to ensure accurate readings.

Voltmeter

This meter measures the potential difference in kV that will be applied to the tube during an exposure. An autotransformer made up of coils with a terminal stud will control the kV. When the switch on the control panel is turned, contact is made with a stud and this will determine the kV selected.

kV compensator

The kV compensator will maintain the kV selected irrespective of the mA selected. The mA must be selected before the kV.

Mains voltage compensation

During the normal working day the mains voltage supply will fluctuate. A lift in the building being used or a lunchtime rush to put all the kettles in the vicinity into use can cause this. The length and width of cables used will also affect the voltage supplied to the unit due to resistance. This must be overcome otherwise the kV selected will be incorrect and the resultant image will be incorrectly exposed. To maintain a constant voltage supply to the X-ray machine, the incoming mains supply is passed over a bank of resistors to give a constant voltage. In some machines this can be altered through the alignment of a needle with a fixed point on a meter. This compensation may be automatic on some larger fixed units.

Operating console

The control panel will have a reading to show the kV selected, another to show the mA or time or mAs selected. The mains voltage compensator selector and reading/indicator will also be found on the control panel. An indication of when an exposure is being made will also be found on the control panel, either in the form of a light or a buzzer. Awareness and familiarity of the operating consol for your particular machine is essential if errors in exposure selection are to be avoided (see Figure 4.8).

Transformers

A transformer is a device for changing an alternating current from one level to another. The transformer is made up of two coils of insulating wire wound onto two metal cores. Each core and winding is separated and insulated so that they form a closed magnetic circuit. Each transformer has several tappings – conductors that end in a terminal stud. A moveable selection switch can make contact with any tapping. In the high-tension circuit the transformer will 'step-up' or increase the voltage. In the filament circuit the transformer will 'step-down' or decrease the voltage. An autotransformer will maintain the voltage at each turn.

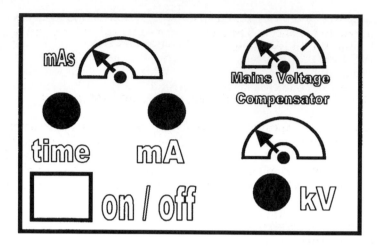

Figure 4.8. Simplified control panel.

Functions of a transformer

- Stabilize mains voltage prior to exposure
- Allow pre-selection of kV
- Supplies voltage to the filament circuit
- Acts as a kV compensator

Filament circuit – control of the mA

The filament circuit will provide the current to the filament in the X-ray tube. This provides the small current (mA) necessary to heat the cathode. Changing the number of resistors that the current flows through alters the filament current. There will be one resistor for each mA value that is available. As the mA increases the temperature of the filament increases, and so the number of electrons available increases.

Space charge compensator

A space charge compensator will maintain the mA irrespective of the kV selected. If this were not present, the alteration of kV would reduce the mA and the number of electrons produced. Radiography needs to be performed using the highest mA possible irrespective of the kV selected and so the space charge compensator is essential.

High-tension circuit – provision of kV

The high-tension circuit provides the kV necessary for an exposure. This usually involves a 1 : 1000 or 1 : 1500 step-up transformer. The kV supplied to the X-ray tube can be adjusted by altering the transformer tappings used.

A rectifier will ensure that the current will only flow in one direction – from the cathode to the anode. The higher the kV selected, the higher the energy levels of the X-rays produced.

Making an exposure – switches, timers and interlocks

The making of an exposure is controlled by the formation and maintenance of a circuit through the X-ray machine. This control can be through switches, timers or interlocks. Whenever an exposure is made there will be a visible or audible (or preferably both) indication that the exposure has been made. This may include movement of the mA indicator, a buzzer or other audible noise.

Primary switching

During an exposure the power will surge. To prevent damage and reverse flow (arcing) through the X-ray tube when the current is applied, switching must be present and accurate. The accuracy of these switches is improved through the use of electromagnets.

Timers

Timers must be accurate, as they will allow the exposure to be made for the required length of time. Exposure will be terminated when the circuit to the tube is opened manually by releasing the exposure button or the timer terminates the exposure. The most basic timer uses a clockwork timer utilizing a tensioned spring that unwinds during the time selected. Electronic timers are more accurate and utilize resistors, smaller resistance for shorter exposure times.

Automatic exposure devices

These are rarely seen in the veterinary field. These devices allow exposure to occur until chambers under the patient detect a pre-selected exposure. At this point the exposure will stop. These systems rely on careful positioning and accurate chamber and exposure selection.

Interlocks

Interlocks will prevent an exposure being made that would result in overheating of the target and subsequent damage. A circuit has a number of switches that open and close the circuit. Unless all of the switches are closed the circuit will not be complete and an exposure will not be possible. Common interlocks include a delay in exposure until the anode is rotating correctly ('prep' stage during exposure process), protection from a very high exposure setting and the prevention of movement of a ceiling suspended tube if there is an obstruction.

Thermal circuit breaker

If the tube and generator overheat, then the circuit will be broken and exposure will be prevented. This happens because the circuit contains a bi-metal strip. This will expand if it heats and the circuit will be broken. The connection will re-form as the strip cools.

Types of X-ray machines

X-ray units fall into a number of distinct categories dependent on their generator type, frequency and mobility.

The main categories are mobile, portable or fixed with distinction made by the amount of movement possible with each machine. Distinction can also be made on the type of generator used and the frequency of the unit. The choice of X-ray machine in the practice will depend on the caseload, the type of examinations expected to be routine and the size and mobility of the unit. The three main types of X-ray machine used in veterinary practice are mobiles, portables and capacitor discharge mobiles. Mobile machines will usually use a 30 A outlet plug.

Some tubes may be mounted to the wall and are described as fixed units. With these machines care should be taken to keep the tracks or runners clean and free from hair that may impair the movement of the machine. They should also be used with a table of a suitable height with a piece of lead rubber to prevent backscatter under the film.

Mobile machine	Motorized, compact, with generator and power supply Mains dependent
Portable machine	Lightweight and compact Low mA
Capacitor discharge	Stores charge until exposure is made 125 kV max 300 mA 1–2 ms to maintain constant potential

Power rating

The power rating of an X-ray machine is described in kW. The standard way of calculating this value is to take the maximum mA possible at 100 kV_p for an exposure of 100 ms to give the maximum available power. This may not be accurate if the X-ray unit uses a single-phase waveform, as the current will fluctuate. The calculation of this rating will not give the rating for the X-ray tube, which may be lower.

Revision points

- The X-ray circuit is made up of the generator, filament circuit, high-tension circuit and the primary circuit
- A generator provides a constant voltage supply to the X-ray machine
- Rectification will provide a current that does not alternate
- Half-wave rectification eliminates the negative part of a waveform
- Full-wave rectification provides a constant positive voltage across the X-ray tube
- Three-phase power provides current that never drops to zero
- High frequency generators provide a near constant waveform with a high frequency
- An X-ray machine can be isolated using the mains supply switch
- The primary circuit contains the meters necessary to determine the exposure factors being set, prior to the exposure being made
- Mains voltage compensation is essential to maintain the voltage at a constant level during an examination
- The operating consol will demonstrate the mains voltage compensation, kV selected; mA and time selected and will provide a local on/off switch
- A transformer will increase or decrease an alternating current
- The filament circuit will control the mA. This will provide the current necessary to heat the cathode
- The high-tension circuit controls the kV supply to the X-ray tube
- Timers will terminate the exposure after a pre-selected period of time
- Interlocks will prevent an exposure being made if the results will damage the X-ray tube or movement of a piece of equipment will cause injury to the operator
- The power rating of an X-ray machine is described in kW

Revision questions

1. *What are the three controls on the X-ray machine control panel?*
2. *What is the first thing you should check when an X-ray machine is switched on?*
3. *On the X-ray machine, which control governs the length of time the X-rays are produced?*
4. *Which of the following statements about X-ray machines is false:*
   (a) Portable machines are high power machines capable of 120mA
   (b) Some mobile machines are battery powered
   (c) The control panel can be some distance from the machine
   (d) Fixed machines can be attached to the ceiling by rails
5. *Portable X-ray machines are low powered machines – this means they have:*
   (a) A low mA output
   (b) A high mA output
   (c) A low kV output
   (d) Mechanical timers
6. *What does a generator do?*
7. *Why is rectification useful in radiography?*
8. *Describe the waveform associated with three-phase power*
9. *How does a transformer work?*
10. *What happens in the filament circuit?*

5 The production of X-rays

Objectives

- The cathode
- The anode
- The X-ray tube
- How X-rays are made
- How to look after your X-ray tube
- Rating your X-ray tube

Introduction

So far, description has examined the processes leading up to the production of X-rays. This chapter looks in detail at the X-ray tube and the actual production of the X-rays. This will include the components of the X-ray tube and the production of X-rays through the interactions of fast moving electrons with the target.

The cathode

The cathode is also known as the filament. The cathode will provide the negative electrode of the X-ray tube that is necessary to allow the electrons to move. The cathode is also the source of electrons necessary for the production of X-rays. The cathode is composed of a wire filament made from tungsten. Tungsten has a high atomic number and very high melting point of 3380°C. The filament of an X-ray tube works in a similar way to the filament in a toaster. In a toaster the filament is heated until it emits heat; in an X-ray tube the filament is heated until it emits electrons. This process of electron production is known as thermionic emission. Using the basic principles described earlier, the use of heat is a very effective method of producing free electrons. Increasing or decreasing the current passing through the filament alters the temperature of the filament. This is through alteration of the mA (Figure 5.1).

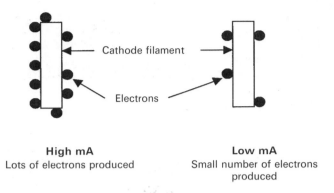

High mA
Lots of electrons produced

Low mA
Small number of electrons produced

Figure 5.1. The effect of mA on electron production.

When the X-ray unit is first switched on the filament is held at a low temperature; the temperature is not high enough for thermionic emission to occur. When the machine is placed in the 'prepare' position the filament is heated to the correct level to allow thermionic emission to produce the necessary electrons. This prevents electron production occurring until the unit is ready for exposures to be made. The temperature of the filament is kept stable during exposure so that the correct number of electrons for the mA selected will be produced.

Cathode	Responsible for electron production
	Composed of the filament and the focusing cup

The focusing cup

The focusing cup contains the filament. All of the electrons are negatively charged and will automatically repel each other. This will mean that the electrons will spread out as they are accelerated towards the anode and some may miss the anode altogether. The focusing cup is negatively charged and will control the electron stream to ensure all electrons strike the anode (see Figure 5.2).

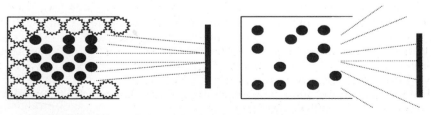

Figure 5.2. The effect of the focusing cup on the electron stream.

Dual-focus tubes

On some machines in use for veterinary work, the focal spot size can be altered. This can be especially useful when examining the main torso of horses and cattle. Focal spot sizes are usually described as fine and broad. The fine focal spot size will provide better resolution to the resultant image with more sharpness caused by a reduction in the penumbra effect (see Figure 5.3).

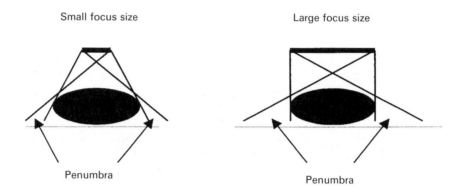

Small focus size   Large focus size

Penumbra   Penumbra

Figure 5.3. Image un-sharpness caused by an increase in focus size.

The reduction in penumbra is due to the smaller size of the electron stream emerging from the focusing cup and striking the anode. The broad focus is especially useful in large animal imaging, as the filament will function with an mA above 400 mA. This will spread the heat on the anode as the electrons strike and allow reduction of the exposure times used.

The length of the filament with fine focus is 0.1–0.5 mm and broad focus is 0.4–1.2 mm. The filament size will however alter from one machine to another.

Fine focus	Small filament size
	Reduction in penumbra
	Good for small animal radiography
Broad focus	Larger filament size
	Higher mA selection possible
	Good for large animal radiography

The anode

The anode is the positive part of the X-ray tube. The anode contains a target that is made from solid tungsten. In machines that are capable of producing multiple exposures with a high exposure the anode will rotate. In these units the tungsten is mounted on molybdenum or graphite to allow easier rotation of the anode.

There are two types of X-ray tube – stationary anode and rotating anode.

Anode	Positive part of the X-ray tube Contains the target that will be struck by electrons to facilitate the production of X-rays

Stationary anode

Stationary anodes are found in portable and some mobile machines where a high tube current and power are not necessary. The anode is fixed in a block of copper to dissipate the heat away from the target. To reduce the heat as much as possible the anode is placed at an angle to the electrons striking the surface. This means that there is a larger area for the electrons to strike while still keeping the focal spot size to a minimum. The angle of the target in a machine with a stationary anode is about $16°$ (see Figure 5.4).

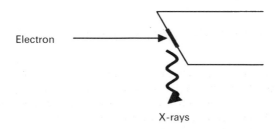

Electron

X-rays

Figure 5.4. Stationary anode.

Rotating anode

This is used in machines that can produce a high output. The anode is in the form of a molybdenum disc with the tungsten anode in the centre in the form of a strip of the element. The anode then rotates at approximately 50 rotations each second and the electrons strike the centre of the strip. This gives a very small focal spot whilst giving a greater area for the heat to be dispersed. This will prevent the pitting and crazing damage that the heat will eventually cause (see Figure 5.5).

Focal Spot	The area on the target being struck by electrons. If the target angle is reduced the focal spot will be reduced
Effective focal spot	This is the size of the focal spot used in the production of a radiographic image

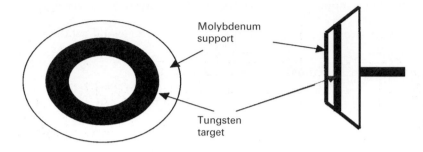

Figure 5.5. Rotating anode.

The X-ray tube

The cathode and anode are contained, supported and protected by the structures known collectively as the X-ray tube. The X-ray tube is supported through the use of fixed or mobile supports. The X-ray tube and its associated supports should never be used to maintain patient position or used as a fixed point when ties are being used (Figure 5.6).

Glass envelope

The anode and cathode are contained within a Pyrex glass envelope. The Pyrex is able to withstand the heat produced during the production of X-rays. This glass envelope has had all the molecules removed to provide a vacuum. The vacuum prevents unwanted collisions occurring before the electrons reach the anode. The cathode and anode are securely fastened to the glass tube to maintain their position. The glass will also insulate the electrodes from each other.

Oil

The glass envelope is surrounded by oil. The oil will take heat away from the tube. The oil will also prevent the tube from overheating. The oil will expand as it heats. A diaphragm within the envelope will move outwards without altering the pressure within the oil. Once the diaphragm reaches its maximum limit a microswitch will be tripped and further X-ray production will be prevented until the oil has cooled and the diaphragm has released the microswitch.

Tube port

The X-rays produced in an X-ray tube will travel in all directions. Only the X-rays that come directly from the target to form the cone of radiation make up the useful beam, otherwise known as the primary beam. The primary beam will pass through the tube port and exit the X-ray tube. The tube port is made of plastic or very thin aluminium. This will absorb all the low energy

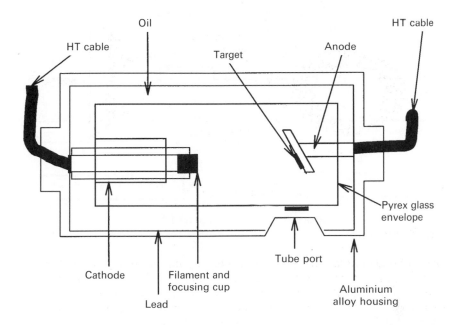

Figure 5.6. Schematic diagram of an X-ray tube.

X-rays that are not useful from the primary beam. All the other X-rays produced will have their path altered or stopped by the lead shielding surrounding the X-ray tube.

Aluminium housing

The aluminium provides a protective housing to help increase the dissipation of heat further. This housing also contains sockets to allow the high-tension cables to make contact with the cathode and the anode. The position of the sockets will alter depending on the movement necessary to use the X-ray tube.

How X-rays are made

The production of X-rays is based on the formation of a current and then the interaction of the electrons in this current with the tungsten target. An mA is applied to the filament at the cathode (negative). This mA will heat the filament and allow electrons to be released. A special focusing cup around the cathode will collect and direct the electrons away from the cathode when the potential difference (kV) is applied between the cathode and the target (focal spot) on the tungsten anode (positive). This occurs within a vacuum so that there are no other particles present to interact with the electrons as they pass across to the anode. As the electrons strike the anode they produce

X-rays. Only 1-5% of the energy of the electron is turned into X-rays, the rest is transformed into heat (see Figure 5.7).

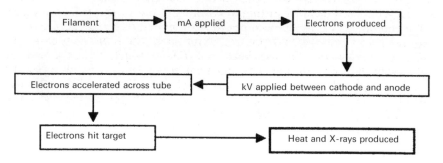

Figure 5.7 The production of X-rays.

How to look after your X-ray tube

Extension of the tube filament life

- Careful selection of mA – consistent use of a very high mA will eventually damage the filament
- Minimizing 'prep' time – when the X-ray tube is in the 'prepare stage', the filament is supplied with a higher current that will evaporate the tungsten
- Minimize careless and rough handling of the tube to protect the filament

Prevention of damage to the anode

- Always remember to warm up your tube with gradually increasing exposure factors before an examination requiring very high exposures is performed. If this is not carried out the high temperature associated with a large exposure may crack the anode.
- Ensure that fine or broad focus is correctly selected to prevent overheating of the anode

General care

- Check for oil leakage on a regular basis to prevent heat damage to the tube.
- Full understanding of the limitations of the machine will extend its life
- Keeping high exposures to a minimum will reduce the tungsten deposits within the tube.
- Choose the tube most suitable for the work you intend to use it for.

Rating your X-ray tube

The tube rating is the maximum amount of electrical energy (the load) that may be applied to the tube by a single exposure, a series of exposures or a single long exposure without causing damage or overheating to any part of the tube assembly. The maximum temperature determines the tube rating each part of its structure can reach before damage will occur. The damage that can be caused includes pitting or cracking of the anode surface, damage to the cathode if the anode becomes too hot and starts to release electrons, melting of the target or the deposition of tungsten within the glass envelope.

Rating is measured in the heat unit (HU), which is calculated by multiplying the kVp with the mAs and a correction factor depending on the generator type. The manufacturer will supply this. The manufacturer will also give details of the maximum load that can be applied by a single exposure using different kV_p values. This is in the form of a chart showing maximum exposure factors at a certain kV_p levels.

Revision points

- The cathode is the negative part of the X-ray tube
- The cathode produces electrons through thermionic emission at the filament
- Electrons are collected in a focusing cup
- The focusing cup will control the electron stream through electrostatic focusing
- The filament size will regulate the size of the focal spot
- The anode is the positive end of the X-ray tube
- The target is made of tungsten
- The target is angled to provide a greater surface area for the electrons to strike
- The cathode and anode are supported in a glass envelope containing a vacuum
- The glass envelope is surrounded by oil, lead and an aluminium casing
- The electrons are accelerated from the cathode to the anode when a potential difference is applied across the tube
- X-rays exit the tube through an opening in the lead that contains aluminium to remove the very low energy X-rays
- Every X-ray tube has a maximum amount of electrical energy it is able to receive known as the tube loading

---

Revision questions

1. Describe the structure of the cathode
2. How is broad and fine focus determined?
3. What function does the focusing cup have?
4. How are the electrons necessary for the production of X-rays produced?
5. What is the difference between a stationary and rotating anode?
6. What is the focal spot?
7. What is the effective focal spot?
8. Give three parts of the tube housing
9. Describe three ways that the X-ray tube can be protected
10. What is the tube rating?

6 The properties of X-rays

Objectives

Characteristic and bremsstrahlung radiation
X-Ray emission spectrum
Altering the emission spectrum
X-Ray quantity
X-Ray quality
The effect on the X-ray beam of striking another atom
Absorption
Attenuation

Introduction

Successful production of X-rays will result in the formation of characteristic radiation. This radiation will have specific properties and will interact with matter in a number of different ways. The interaction will depend on the material and the velocity of the X-ray at the time of the interaction.

Characteristic and bremsstrahlung radiation

When an X-ray is first produced a process called bremsstrahlung occurs as the electron decelerates to produce an X-ray photon. This is sometimes known as braking radiation. As an electron comes near the nucleus of an atom in the target, it will slow down and change course. During this time it will lose kinetic energy. This loss in kinetic energy will appear as an X-ray. The X-rays produced in this way can be of different energy levels and the interaction will occur randomly. The energy formed cannot be greater than the kV_p selected.

   The production of characteristic radiation (Figure 6.1) occurs in a similar way, but the X-rays produced will be of a specific energy level. This occurs when the electron from an inner shell is ejected from the atom and an outer shell electron falls into the empty space created. As this outer shell electron moves, an X-ray is emitted. The energy of the X-rays produced will be equal to the energy binding the electrons involved together.

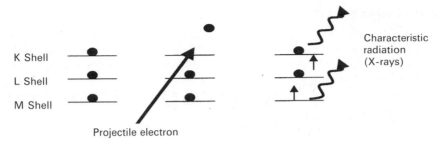

K Shell

L Shell

M Shell

Projectile electron

Characteristic
radiation
(X-rays)

Figure 6.1. The production of characteristic radiation.

X-Ray emission spectrum

The X-ray emission spectrum is a demonstration of the energy of each
individual X-ray produced during an exposure. In the emission spectrum the
number of X-rays produced is plotted against the energy of each individual
X-ray photon. The X-ray spectrum is specific to the type of machine and will
alter depending on the type of photon being measured. Changing the kV_p,
mA, time and inherent filtration of the machine can alter the spectrum.

Characteristic X-ray spectrum

Characteristic radiation will produce a line spectrum. All of the units will
have fixed values that are specific to each individual element. Tungsten will
have 15 energy levels. These are demonstrated as straight lines on the
emission spectrum, one line for each electron shell of the atom. These are as
K or L X-rays depending on the shell that the electrons have been ejected
from and the relative energy levels. These are the thin lines in Figure 6.2. L
lines will not be represented if the tube output is demonstrated. This is
because the soft radiation will have been removed through the aluminium
filtration present.

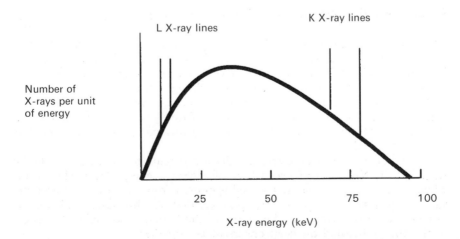

L X-ray lines

K X-ray lines

Number of
X-rays per unit
of energy

25   50   75   100

X-ray energy (keV)

Figure 6.2. Characteristic and bremsstrahlung emission spectrum.

Bremsstrahlung X-ray spectrum

The formation of X-rays through bremsstrahlung will produce a continuous spectrum. This will extend from zero to the maximum energy possessed by the electrons. The majority of X-rays (producing a peak) will have about one third of the maximum energy. This is the thicker curved line in Figure 6.2.

Altering the emission spectrum

A number of different factors will alter the emission spectrum. If these alterations are understood, then the effects on the resultant image can be understood.

Change in atomic number

The intensity of X-rays produced is directly proportional to the atomic number of the target. If the atomic number is low, then the number of X-rays produced will be lower. The k lines will move to a lower photon energy level. The maximum photon energy and spectrum shape will remain unchanged (see Figure 6.3).

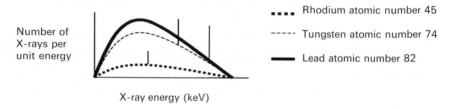

Figure 6.3. The effect of atomic number on emission spectrum.

Change in mA

The mA is directly proportional to the number of X-rays produced. If the mA is doubled, then twice as many electrons will be produced at the cathode with the result of twice as many X-rays being produced for each energy level. The maximum energy levels will, however, remain the same. The k lines will remain at the same energy level (see Figure 6.4).

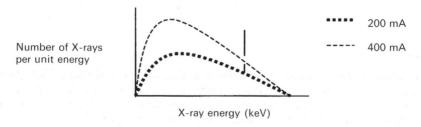

Figure 6.4. The effect of mA on emission spectrum.

Change in kV$_p$

The intensity of X-rays is directly proportional to the square of the kV. If the kV$_p$ is increased, then far more electrons are released from the cathode and so the number of X-rays at each energy level will increase dramatically. This increase will be greater at the higher energy levels. The maximum energy level will also increase. If the kV$_p$ is decreased the spectral peak will move to a lower value and the k radiation may not be produced (see Figure 6.5).

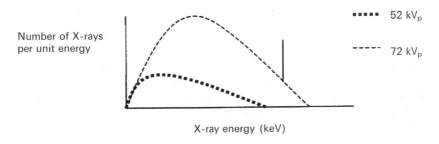

Figure 6.5. The effect of changing the kV$_p$ on emission spectrum.

> Increasing the kV$_p$ by 15% is equal to doubling the mAs for a given optical density

Effect of waveform

If the X-ray unit uses a high frequency or three-phase power source, then there will be a higher number of X-rays for each energy level. A machine using three-phase power will be more efficient than a single-phase power machine. Different types of rectification do not alter the emission spectrum.

> Three-phase power is equivalent to a 12% increase in kV$_p$ or double the mAs in a single-phase machine

Effect of filtration

Alteration in the filtration of the beam will alter the spectral shape. Filtration will remove the low energy photons from the beam and move the peak to a higher energy level. There will also be a reduction in the intensity, but the maximum photon energy will remain the same (see Figure 6.6).

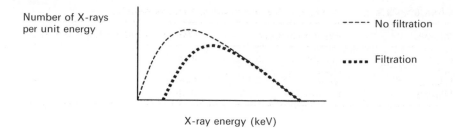

Number of X-rays per unit energy

- - - - No filtration

..... Filtration

X-ray energy (keV)

Figure 6.6. The effect of filtration on the emission spectrum.

Atomic number	↑	More X-rays produced for each energy level, higher peak energy level
mA	↑	More X-rays produced for each energy level
kV	↑	Higher peak energy level, more X-rays for each energy level produced
Filtration		Filtration will remove low energy level X-rays, peak energy level will be lower
Waveform		High-frequency machines will have a higher number of X-rays produced for each energy level

X-Ray quantity

The quantity of X-rays produced or the intensity is the description of the number of X-rays in the useful beam. The useful beam is the beam that forms the radiographic image. The X-ray quantity can be calculated by monitoring the rate of flow of energy through a unit area at right angles to the beam.

The alteration of mAs, kV_p, distance and filtration will all alter the density of the resultant image (optical density). Increasing or decreasing these factors will all increase or decrease the optical density in a similar direction, although the changes may not be of a similar size. The calculation of the new and old factors is discussed in a later chapter.

X-Ray quality

The X-ray quality describes the penetrating power of the beam. This is measured in terms of the half value layer. This is the thickness of material that reduces the intensity of the beam to half of its original intensity. This is affected by the kV_p and the filtration used. If the kV is high, the X-rays will penetrate the object being radiographed further than softer, low energy X-rays. The high kV X-rays will have a greater have value layer (see Table 6.1).

Table 6.1. Effects on X-ray quality and resultant image density

Increase	Effect on quality	Effect on resultant image density
kV$_p$	Increase	Increase
mAs	None	Increase
Distance	None	Reduce
Filtration	Increase	Reduce

The effect of the X-ray beam striking another atom

All X-rays will interact with matter to produce secondary radiation. Secondary radiation is any radiation produced by an object that has been radiated. This radiation will travel in any direction and is described as scatter. The amount of scattered radiation will depend on the density of the patient and the atomic number of the tissues. If the tissues contain elements with high atomic numbers or the patient is large, scatter will be increased. As the size of the field increases, the amount of scatter will increase so limitation of the primary beam can be used to reduce scattered radiation. As is already known, as the kV$_p$ increases, the wavelength of the primary beam will increase. This will give the primary beam and the secondary radiation more penetrating power, and results in more scattered radiation reaching the film. The scattered radiation caused by a patient can be reduced through the use of a grid, discussed later, or the use of a compression band. A compression band will reduce the volume of tissue in a given area and will reduce the exposure necessary. This in turn will reduce the kV needed and will increase the contrast of the resultant image. In veterinary work, placing a patient in dorsal or ventral recumbency can reduce the volume of tissue to improve contrast in very large or obese animals. In diagnostic radiography only the Compton effect and photoelectric absorption will have an effect on the types of scattered radiation produced. The Compton effect will result in no diagnostic information reaching the film and photoelectric absorption results in all the X-ray photons being absorbed. Only X-ray photons that pass through the patient without interacting will produce a diagnostic image.

Classical scattering

Classical scattering is not particularly important in radiography. If the X-ray photon has a low energy level in comparison to the binding energy of the electrons in the matter it will interact with electrons in the outer shells. This will make the electrons vibrate. The X-ray photon emitted will have the same energy level as the incident photon but will be moving in a different direction.

Photoelectric absorption

Photoelectric absorption will result in the X-ray photon being totally absorbed by the matter. The X-ray photon interacts with a bound electron as long as the energy of the incoming photon is equal to or greater than the binding energy of the electron. The ejected electron will have kinetic energy that is equal to the binding energy of the incident photon. The ejected electron will travel through matter losing energy. The atom is left in an excited state. An electron falling from an outer shell into the inner shell, filling the gap fills the vacancy. The energy given off during this movement is emitted as characteristic radiation (see Figure 6.7).

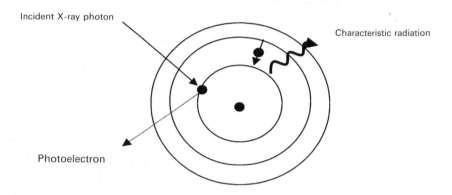

Figure 6.7. The process of photoelectric absorption.

Compton effect

The Compton effect will occur when the X-ray photon interacts with a free electron. The energy of the incident photon is shared between the electron and the scattered photon. The photon can be scattered anywhere from 0° to 180°. The electron will always be scattered forwards. This is known as the scatter angle. If the angle of scatter is small then the photon has lost energy and the electron has received energy. This type of scattering is not related to atomic number but does depend on the density of electrons present (see Figure 6.8).

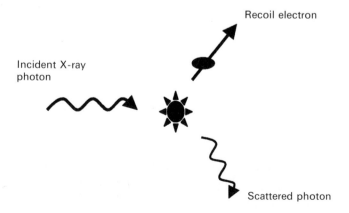

Figure 6.8. The Compton effect.

Absorption

During absorption, the energy from the X-ray photon is transferred to the atoms of the absorber. As more energy is absorbed, the lower the number of X-ray photons passing through the matter and forming the image on the film. This absorption can be as a result of the energy of the X-ray photons or the atomic number of the matter. During absorption the photoelectric effect will be taking place (see Figure 6.9).

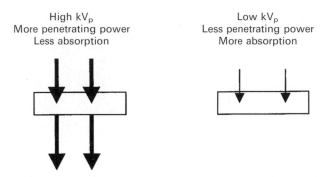

High kV_p
More penetrating power
Less absorption

Low kV_p
Less penetrating power
More absorption

Figure 6.9. The effect of kV_p on the absorption of an X-ray photon.

Attenuation

Attenuation is the reduction in intensity of the X-ray beam as it passes through matter. This can be due to absorption or scatter or a combination of both. Every type of matter will have a different attenuation coefficient. This is the effectiveness of the matter to attenuate or absorb the radiation passing through. Every X-ray will have a fixed range through tissue; this will depend on the atomic number of the atoms involved and the density of the atoms within the tissue. Attenuation is the sum of the X-ray photons scattered and absorbed.

Attenuation = absorption + scatter

Revision points

- Characteristic radiation occurs when an electron interacts with an inner shell electron at the target – as the inner shell space is filled, characteristic radiation is released
- Bremsstrahlung radiation is produced as the electron is stopped at the target – this electron will loose kinetic energy
- Bremsstrahlung radiation is the type most commonly formed during the use of an X-ray tube using diagnostic-level exposures
- X-ray emission spectra demonstrate the energy level of each X-ray photon produced during an exposure
- Characteristic radiation will produce discrete lines
- Bremsstrahlung radiation will produce a curve
- Characteristic spectra can be altered by changing the mA, kV_p, target material, voltage waveform or by adding filtration
- X-ray quantity can be increased by increasing the mAs, kV_p or the atomic number of the target material or decreased by increasing the filtration used or the voltage waveform used
- X-ray quality can be increased by increasing the kV_p and the filtration used
- X-ray quality is described as the half value layer – the amount of material needed to reduce the X-ray beam by half
- Classical scattering is a change in the direction of the X-ray photon without a loss in energy
- Compton effect is caused when the incident X-ray photon ionizes the atom and the X-ray changes direction and looses energy
- Photoelectric absorption occurs when the X-ray photon is absorbed by one of the electrons in the inner shell of the atom; a photoelectron is emitted with an energy level nearly equal to that of the incident X-ray photon; characteristic radiation is also emitted as the inner shell fills
- Attenuation is the reduction in the intensity of an X-ray beam as it passes through matter
- Attenuation is the sum of absorption and scatter

Revision questions

1. *Describe the production of bremsstrahlung radiation*
2. *Is characteristic radiation produced during a diagnostic examination?*
3. *Draw a diagram of an emission spectrum*
4. *How can the emission spectrum be altered? Give four factors*
5. *What percentage change of kV_p is equal to doubling the mAs?*
6. *Describe X-ray quantity*
7. *What factors can alter the X-ray quantity?*
8. *What is X-ray quality?*
9. *How is X-ray quality measured?*
10. *Give two factors that will alter X-ray quality*
11. *Describe the Compton effect*
12. *Describe photoelectric absorption*
13. *What is the relationship between the density of a material and the absorption of X-rays?*
14. *What is attenuation?*
15. *What is attenuation equal to?*

Intensifying screens and cassettes

Objectives

- The construction of intensifying screens
- Luminescence
- Film–screen combinations
- Film–screen contact
- Care of intensifying screens
- Construction of cassettes
- Care and use of cassettes

Introduction

Intensifying screens are found within the cassette used for radiographic examinations. The screen will convert the energy from the X-ray beam into light and this light will expose the film. This will reduce the exposure necessary to produce a diagnostic radiograph and at the same time improving radiation safety. Less than 1% of the X-ray beam actually exposes the radiographic film, the remainder of the exposure coming from the light emitted from intensifying screens.

The construction of intensifying screens

Intensifying screens are constructed in sizes to be used with the corresponding cassette size. Radiographic film is sandwiched between a pair of intensifying screens inside the cassette. If two screens are to be used, double-emulsion film is used. If more detail is required a single screen can be used. If a single screen is to be used, a single-emulsion film will be necessary. The emulsion side of the film should be in contact with the intensifying screen.

The screen is composed of four distinct parts: the protective coating, phosphor layer, reflective layer and the base (see Figure 7.1).

Protective coating

The outer layer of the intensifying screen is the protective coating made from acetate. This is the part of the screen in contact with the X-ray film. It will

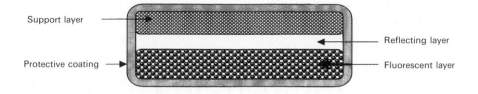

Support layer

Reflecting layer

Protective coating

Fluorescent layer

Figure 7.1. Cross-sectional view of an intensifying screen.

protect the screen against abrasions, moisture and staining. The coating will also reduce static electricity that may cause an artefact. The protective coating can undergo routine cleaning without any damage if strict guidelines are followed. This layer extends around the back of the screen where it provides a non-curl backing.

Reflecting layer

The reflective layer is made of either magnesium oxide or titanium dioxide. This layer will redirect light emitted in a direction that will not expose the film. This will increase the function of the intensifying screen. Some intensifying screens may contain dyes that will absorb this stray light. This will prevent image blur, but will not improve the function of the intensifying screen.

Base

The base is at the back of the intensifying screen. This acts as a support for the screen. It is made of either high-grade cardboard or polyester. These materials are usually selected as they provide a strong moisture resistant material, whilst remaining flexible. The base must also not react with the phosphor layer or be visible on the resultant image.

Fluorescent phosphor layer

This is the layer within the intensifying screen that is active. It contains a layer of tiny phosphor crystals suspended in a binder of polyurethane. The binder holds the crystals together and prevents moisture affecting the crystals. The binder also contains a coloured pigment or carbon granules that function in a similar way to the dye in the reflective layer. The combination and proportions of these components will determine the speed of the intensifying screen.

The phosphors selected must be very good at absorbing X-rays and must fluoresce well with some afterglow. This afterglow is not used in radiography and will not be described any further. The two main types of phosphors used are either from the rare earth group or calcium tungstate. Rare earth intensifying screens are more effective than calcium tungstate at changing X-ray photons to light (15–20% efficiency compared to 3–5% efficiency with calcium tungstate). Some rare earth screens will have an impurity added to alter the colour of light emitted and the intensity of the light. The rare earth screens contain oxysulphides of gadolinium, lanthanum, yttrium or any of the other elements from the rare earth group of the periodic table. Calcium tungstate was the original phosphor used for radiography and emits blue light.

Luminescence

Luminescence can be separated into two separate categories – fluorescence and phosphorescence. Both occur when a phosphor is bombarded by radiation, in radiography the radiation is in the form of X-rays. Fluorescence is the emission of the light during exposure whereas phosphorescence is the afterglow.

Fluorescence occurs when X-ray photons pass through the phosphor layer of the intensifying screen. The phosphor crystal absorbs the X-ray photon. This phosphor becomes excited emitting ultraviolet and visible light. This visible light is used to make the latent image on a radiographic film (see Figure 7.2).

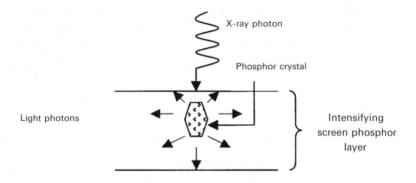

Figure 7.2. Luminescence.

The phosphor will emit hundreds of light photons for every X-ray photon that strikes it. This is why, along with the fact that radiographic film is more sensitive to light, less exposure is necessary to provide an image if an intensifying screen is used.

Film–screen combinations

To ensure that the best is made of the screens and the film available a number of factors need to be considered.

Light emission and film selection

The colour emitted from the screen needs to be matched with the colour sensitivity of the film. If the screen phosphor emits green light, then it should be used with orthochromatic film. This ensures that point of maximum sensitivity of the film will match the screen maximum light emission. This means that the optimum speed for the system will be obtained. If the film sensitivity is not matched to the light emitted from the screens, then the effects of using the intensifying screen will be reduced (see Table 7.1).

Table 7.1. Film–screen combinations

Phosphor type	Colour emitted from screen	Colour sensitivity of film
Calcium tungstate	Blue	Blue (monochromatic)
Rare earth	Green (sometimes blue)	Blue or green (orthochromatic)

Speed

Intensifying screens are usually divided in to three categories – slow, medium and fast (Table 7.2). The distinction between the categories will depend on the intensification factor or the exposure required to produce a suitable, diagnostic image using intensifying screens. The screens usually come in pairs of similar speeds although the screen placed on the back of the cassette will have a thicker layer of phosphors. This ensures that the film is evenly exposed. Uneven exposure may occur, as the X-rays reaching the second screen will have passed through the film and front screen, losing energy on the way. This may reduce the light emitted from each phosphor, reducing the exposure to the film.

Table 7.2. Screen speeds

Screen	Speed	Uses
High resolution	Slow	Fine detail, needs higher exposure so should be used where lower exposure factors are acceptable
Regular	Medium	General radiography
Fast	Fast	Produce a darker radiographic image for given exposure factors when compared to regular or high resolution screens; Ideal for use where movement may be a problem

The speed of screen can be altered by the phosphor grain size, the thickness of the intensifying layer, the presence or absence of a reflective layer and the amount of crossover that may occur from screen to film.

Speed	Relative exposures needed by different intensifying screens to produce an image of similar density
	Faster screens require less exposure to produce a similar image to a medium or slow screen

Single-screen use

A single screen can be used with specifically produced films. The screen is placed at the back of the cassette to prevent unnecessary divergence of the light prior to reaching the film emulsion. This will improve the sharpness of the resultant image. This type of screen will improve image quality and sharpness, but will require a high exposure to produce a diagnostic image.

Assessing the speed of a new film–screen combination

Every intensifying screen and film combination will require specific exposure factors. If a new set of screens or film is used the change in speed can be assessed by imaging either a step wedge or a specimen using both combinations (new and old). This will demonstrate the changes necessary in exposure factor to produce a similar radiographic density.

Quantum mottle

If a very fast film–screen combination is used with low exposure factors, quantum mottle may occur. This appears as a mottled or even spotty appearance to the resultant image. This occurs if there are not enough photons of light to produce an image on the film. This may be due to the inability of the film to detect the small amount of light or the lack of light produced in the first instance from the intensifying screens.

Film–screen contact

Contact between the screens and film is essential if a high-quality or sharp radiograph is to be obtained. If the contact between the film and screens is not even areas of the radiograph will appear blurred and un-sharp. This effect will occur as the light has spread out through divergence before coming into contact with the film emulsion. Divergence from a number of phosphor crystals may overlap to increase the un-sharpness further. Poor film–screen contact can be assessed by placing a wire mesh (metal strip with sequins removed is adequate) on top of the cassette and producing a radiograph. If there is poor contact the edges of the circles will be fuzzy and not sharp.

Care of intensifying screens

Any intensifying screen that is damaged cannot be repaired and is useless for the function it was intended. If one screen becomes damaged, it is usually necessary to replace both screens. The function of the screen can be impaired by dust, foreign matter such as animal hair, finger marks or stains. Care should be taken not to touch the screens unnecessarily or leave the cassettes open longer than is necessary as this increases the chances of spillage occurring or something being dropped directly onto the screen. The screens are very sensitive to moisture and temperature, so careful consideration should be given to their storage.

Cleaning screens

Screens should be cleaned regularly to remove any dust or other foreign material from their surfaces. This can be done easily using a mild liquid detergent or a proprietary screen cleaner.

- A soft cloth, but not cotton wool (as it leaves tiny fibres) should be moistened with the detergent and wiped gently over the screen
- The screen should never become wet and spillage to the back of the screen must be avoided
- The screen should then be wiped clean using a fresh dry cloth or piece of gauze
- The cassette should then be left standing upright and slightly open to allow it to dry
- It is a good idea to record when this is done.

Construction of cassettes

The screens and film of choice are contained within a cassette. This will protect them from damage and prevent dust accumulation on the screens. The cassette will also maintain close contact between the film and screens, and also prevent light reaching the film and causing fogging. The insides of all cassettes are black to prevent the reflection of internal light.

Cassette front

The front of the cassette is a uniform thickness and should conform to British Standards (BS 4304/1968). If the cassette is plastic it should have an aluminium equivalent of no more than 0.2 mm. This will minimize the attenuation of the beam. The front is usually made from plastic or carbon fibre. This provides stiffness whilst still being lightweight. The materials used will also have a low absorption of the beam. Carbon fibre will reduce patient dose especially at lower kV levels. The front of the cassette will also incorporate a recessed well that will contain the screen and a lead strip to block radiation. This allows for patient identification.

Cassette back

The back is usually of a similar material to the front and is lined with lead foil to protect the film from backscatter. The back is usually curved to ensure good film screen contact. The back may also contain a foam pressure pad under the intensifying screen to increase film screen contact further.

Closure

All cassettes have a method of ensuring that the cassette remains closed and that adequate film–screen contact is maintained. These methods range from spring clips made of metal to plastic locking bars and plastic clips.

Care and use of cassettes

Cassettes can be damaged and care should be taken.

- Use them gently
- Do not drop them
- Carry a few at a time
- Cassettes can be damaged if they are stored at an angle so they should be as near to vertical as possible
- If the cassette is used under a patient, the use of a cassette tunnel should be considered to prevent unnecessary pressure being applied to the cassette
- Try to avoid getting the cassettes wet – if this is unavoidable, cover the cassette in a waterproof covering (a carrier bag is adequate!)
- Number all cassettes, and keep a record of their first use, any damage that occurs and any maintenance that is carried out

---

Revision points

- An intensifying screen will convert X-rays into light
- An intensifying screen will reduce the patient dose
- Intensifying screens are composed of a layer of phosphor crystals in a binder
- The phosphor layer is covered in a protective coating
- The main categories of intensifying screens are either rare earth or fast tungstate
- The intensification factor is the exposure required to produce a satisfactory image using intensifying screens
- Screens have three speeds – slow, medium and fast
- The faster an intensifying screen, the lower the exposure necessary to produce a diagnostic image
- Film screen contact must be good to prevent a loss in detail
- Screens must be protected from scratches, chemical splashes and moisture
- Cassettes contain the film and screens
- The cassette will maintain good film screen contact and will prevent light from reaching the film
- The cassette is usually made of plastic or carbon fibre
- The cassette should have low beam absorption

Revision questions

1. Describe the function of an intensifying screen
2. How does a phosphor grain convert X-rays into light?
3. Name the three speeds of screen and when each may be used
4. What are the two main types of phosphor used in an intensifying screen?
5. Give two factors that can alter the speed of a screen
6. Why is film screen contact so essential?
7. How would you clean a screen?
8. Describe the layers within an X-ray cassette
9. Why are the insides of a cassette black?
10. Give three main points to consider when caring for a cassette

8 Radiographic film

Objectives

- Film construction
- Types of film
- Care and storage of films
- Formation of the latent image
- Film sensitivity
- Duplication film

Introduction

The production of a radiograph relies upon the exposure of a patient to radiation, but also to the formation of a latent image either on a radiographic film that can be viewed at a later date or more recently in the form of a digital image. This chapter will examine the 'make-up' of a radiographic film and the formation of a latent image that will form the permanent image during development. At the present time digital imaging is beyond the financial scope of most veterinary practices and will be briefly discussed in the chapter on alternative imaging techniques (Chapter 13).

Film construction

Radiographic film is constructed of a number of distinct layers all with specific functions. Whether film is duplitized (two emulsion sides) or is single-sided, it will have a base layer, a subbing layer, an emulsion and a supercoat to protect the emulsion. If the film is duplitized, the layers will be duplicated on the reverse side of the base. If the film is single-sided, it will have an anti-halation layer and an anti-curl layer on the reverse side of the base (see Figure 8.1).

Film base

The film base provides a support for the emulsion and is usually transparent to transmitted light when the radiograph is being reviewed. Polyester is usually the chosen compound as it strong, flexible and chemically inert. It

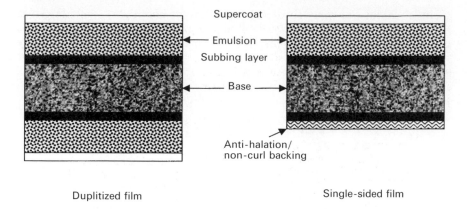

Supercoat

Emulsion

Subbing layer

Base

Anti-halation/
non-curl backing

Duplitized film   Single-sided film

Figure 8.1. Cross-section through duplitized and single-sided emulsion film.

will maintain its shape and form despite changes in moisture and temperature. Polyester can be produced to a uniform thickness so an even coating of the emulsion is possible. This is essential, as varying thicknesses of emulsion will result in an uneven image. The base usually has a blue dye added at manufacture and this colour will remain consistent from one batch to another. The film base is usually 0.18 mm thick.

Subbing layer

The subbing layer is composed of gelatine and reactive ester salts. The subbing layer forms an adhesive for the emulsion. If the subbing layer was not used the emulsion would peel away from the base when it was dry and form a layer of sludge when it was wet. Some manufacturers add a dye to prevent cross-over from occurring.

> Cross-over occurs when light passes from one screen, through the film and exposes the opposing side of the film – this light is travelling a larger distance than normal and will result in greater divergence and un-sharpness

Emulsion

The emulsion contains the active part of the film. The emulsion is made up of gelatine with small crystals of silver halides suspended throughout. Gelatine is used as it can exist as a liquid or a solid, and can be applied to the film base easily and evenly as a liquid and can then become a solid suitable for storage and use. The gelatine is permeable to water and will allow the processing chemicals access to the silver halide crystals. The gelatine will also keep the grains separated to prevent clumping and uneven distribution of the silver halide grains. The silver halide grains may be either tabular or globular. The globular grains are monochromatic (sensitive to blue light), tabular grains are orthochromatic or sensitive to blue and green light. The tabular grains are a particular shape depending on their manufacture and will fit closely together giving increased resolution, less cross-over and a greater light absorption. Grain size and shape will also enhance the image quality due to changes in the amounts of un-sharpness caused by the grains (see Figure 8.2).

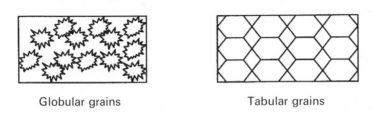

Globular grains   Tabular grains

Figure 8.2. Film coverage of globular and tabular grains.

Some emulsions will be sensitized to prevent certain colours of light from passing through. The silver halide is manufactured within the gelatine following a reaction of silver nitrate and a halide compound. This technique is used to ensure that the silver halide is not exposed to any radiation prior to use. If the film is duplitized the emulsion will be applied to both sides of the base. If the film is single-sided only one emulsion layer will be added to the base. In single-sided and direct exposure film the emulsion will be thicker than that found on duplitized film.

Supercoat

The supercoat is a very thin layer of gelatine that will protect the film during processing and during handling after processing. The surface is semi-matt to help the rollers in the processor to move the film.

Anti-halation/curl layer

This layer is found in single-sided film. As the film is processed the emulsion swells and this will cause the base to curl. In duplitized film the two emulsion layers will counteract each other. In single-sided films the second side is coated with a layer of gelatine to prevent the film from curling.

A dye is also added to the backing to prevent scattered light reflected from the base of the film influencing the true image. This reflection is known as halation. The colour of this dye will vary depending on the colour sensitivity of the film (see Figure 8.3).

Light from intensifying screen

Scattered light
reflected back
from the base
causing
un-sharpness

Light absorbed by anti-
halation backing

Figure 8.3. Effect of an anti-halation layer.

Types of film

Screen film

Screen film is designed to be used in conjunction with intensifying screens. The image on the film will be formed through direct exposure to X-rays, but mainly through light emitted from the phosphors on the screens. The use of two screens will double the efficiency of the X-ray beam and reduce the exposure required.

There are two main types of radiographic film in use – duplitized and single-sided film. Duplitized film has two emulsions which reduces the number of X-rays necessary to produce a diagnostic image. This will lessen the wear on the X-ray tube and will increase the contrast on the film. Single-sided screen film has one emulsion layer which reduces cross-over and parallax, giving a more detailed image. This increased detail is at the cost of a reduction of exposure and image contrast.

Non-screen film

This type of film relies on direct exposure to produce an image. It is used in human dental radiography and mainly in intra-oral examinations of the nasal chambers in the veterinary field. The emulsion layer is thicker so that more silver halide crystals are present to form the latent image. This type of film gives greater detail but requires a much higher exposure (typically 5–25 times the exposure necessary for normal screen radiography). Larger non-screen film suitable for intra-oral examinations are difficult to obtain, and so single-sided film cut to size and placed in a light tight envelope can be used. Due to the thickened emulsion and enlarged grain size, this type of film will require longer processing times than screen film.

Radiation monitoring film

This type of film is similar to non-screen film in appearance. Although it is duplitized, it has different speeds of emulsion on each side. This ensures that a wide range of exposure levels can be recorded and monitored. If a large exposure is received the whole film may be black with a fast emulsion, but this can be removed to demonstrate the density of the slower emulsion giving an accurate estimation of the dose received.

Polaroid film

This type of film uses a special light sensitive negative sheet in an envelope that is exposed to X-rays and light from a single screen. This is then processed in a special unit with a transparent blue-tinted polyester positive imaging sheet and processing chemicals. The positive image is viewed after processing. This is of use for equine work where the darkroom may be some distance from the examination area.

Care and storage of films

Film is sensitive to light, radiation and moisture, and so the film needs to be stored to prevent damage from any of these factors. The film is well packaged by the manufacturers and so the film should be kept in this packaging until ready for use.

Expiry dates and stock rotation

A careful note of the expiry date should be made and older stock should be used first. Storage of film is not ideal over longer periods of time and so small regular orders of film mean that it will be in better condition when it is needed.

Protection of the film

Under pressure or rough handling the emulsion can be damaged and artefacts will be seen on the resultant image. Films should be stored vertically to prevent the pressure from other boxes damaging the film.

The film is also sensitive to damp and moisture and so the room used for storage should be dry and cool with good ventilation. If the room temperature drops below 15°C then the box should be brought back to room temperature slowly before use.

Care should be taken to avoid storing the film in the same room as the X-ray equipment or next door to the X-ray room if a horizontal beam is used. Any exposure to radiation will result in fogging of the film.

The film should also be stored away from certain chemicals and fumes, especially those found in the processing chemistry.

Storage of opened boxes

Once opened, boxes of films should be stored in either a specially designed film hopper or in a light tight drawer. The film should remain in the boxes with the internal wrappings folded over and the lid on securely.

Formation of the latent image

The formation of a latent image is a series of steps involving the interaction of light or X-rays with a silver halide crystal. The silver and bromine atoms are fixed in a lattice. Each crystal is charged, as the silver will lose an electron to form a bond with the bromine. The atom is not rigid and so the silver ions will be found within the crystal while the negatively charged bromine atoms will be found on the surface of the crystal.

Silver halide reaction

The interaction of light or X-rays with the crystal will result in the release of electrons. The electron will migrate to the sensitivity speck within the crystal. This will allow the formation of metallic silver at the sensitivity speck with negative bromine atoms being released. The will be repeated every time the crystal is exposed to light. Eventually the negative surface charge of the bromine will disappear and the amount of silver in the crystal will increase. This collection of silver atoms is the latent image. The remaining silver halide will be converted during processing to a visible image (see Figure 8.4).

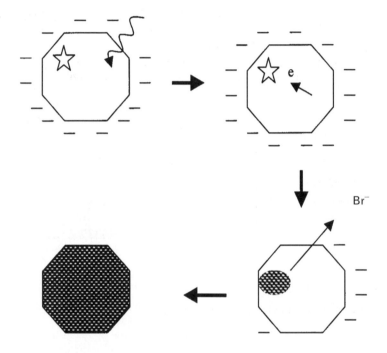

Figure 8.4. The silver halide reaction.

Film sensitivity

It is already known that X-ray film is more sensitive to the light from intensifying screen than X-rays alone. Light is made up of different colours and the emulsion will react differently to the component colours of light. This response can be controlled by the addition of dyes during manufacture. Without a sensitizer the emulsion is more sensitive to blue, violet and ultraviolet light. This type of emulsion is known as monochromatic film. If the sensitizer is present, then the range of colour sensitivity can be increased to include green light. This film is known as orthochromatic. Some film sensitivity can be increased to include red light. This type of film is described as panchromatic.

A graph can be plotted to demonstrate the sensitivity of the film (speed) against the wavelength of light that it is exposed to.

Film speed	The sensitivity of film to light or radiation – fast films require less exposure to give a similar film using a slow film

Sensitivity is calculated and assessed by measurement of the densities produced when a film is subjected to different wavelengths of light for equal exposure times. This curve will determine the film screen combination possible and the type of safelight needed in the darkroom to protect the film from exposure. Peak sensitivity is always shown as 1 (see Figure 8.5).

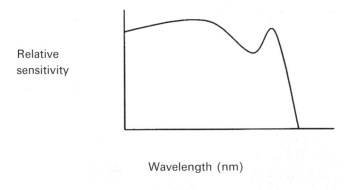

Relative sensitivity

Wavelength (nm)

Figure 8.5. Sensitivity curve of a common orthochromatic film.

Duplicating film

Radiographs can be copied using a special film. This type of film starts as black when viewed unexposed and developed. If the radiograph to be copied is placed in close contact with this type of film and exposed to white or ultraviolet light from a light source a copy will be obtained from the original (see Figure 8.6).

During the copying process, light passes through the translucent parts of the original radiograph and will expose the duplicating film. Light cannot penetrate the blackened parts of the original film so the duplicating film will remain un-exposed and will remain or appear black on processing.

This type of film is single-sided. The density of the film will reduce with increasing exposure, the reverse to normal film. If a duplicated film appears underexposed the time of exposure to light needs to be reduced.

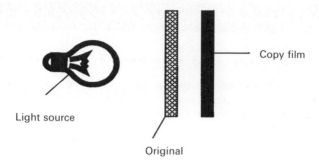

Figure 8.6. Contact copying of radiographs.

Revision points

- Film is made up of distinct layers
- The base is made of polyester and supports the emulsion
- The subbing layer is composed of gelatine and forms an adhesive for the emulsion
- The emulsion is made up of gelatine with silver halide grains in suspension
- The gelatine prevents the silver halide grains from bunching
- Grains of silver halide may be globular or tabular
- Emulsion can be sensitized using dyes to different wavelengths of light
- The supercoat is a very thin layer of gelatine that will protect the film during processing and storage
- In single-sided films an anti-halation layer and curl layer is placed on the reverse of the base.
- Screen film is designed to be used in conjunction with intensifying screens
- Duplitized film has emulsion on both sides and is used with two screens
- Non-screen film is exposed using X-rays alone
- Non-screen film requires 5–25 times more exposure than screen film
- Radiation monitoring film is duplitized but has emulsions of different speeds
- Polaroid film can be used where no processing facilities are available
- Films should be stored upright in a dry, cool room with good ventilation
- Film boxes should not be stacked as the film is sensitive to pressure
- Film should be used in date order
- The latent image is formed though the interaction of light with the silver halide crystal in the emulsion
- Film sensitivity is sometimes described as the speed of a film
- A film with a high speed will require less exposure than a slower film to produce an image of a similar density
- Film duplication uses a special film that works in reverse to a conventional film

Revision questions

1. *Draw a diagram of a duplitized film*
2. *What are the structural differences between duplitized and single-sided film?*
3. *Why is gelatine used as the support for the silver halide crystals in the emulsion?*
4. *How is the emulsion of a film sensitized?*
5. *What is halation?*
6. *Why should an animal be anaesthetized when using a non-screen film?*
7. *When would Polaroid film be useful?*
8. *How should radiographic film be stored?*
9. *Outline the four stages of the silver halide reaction*
10. *What is film speed?*

9 Forming the visible image

Objectives

- The steps of processing
- Developing
- Fixing
- Washing
- Drying
- Developer solution
- Fixer solution
- Control of Substances Hazardous to Health Regulations (COSHH)

Introduction

Once the latent image has been formed on the emulsion layer of the radiographic film, development must take place so that the visible image may be appreciated. The process of producing this image is called development. Development is one of the areas where unacceptable radiographs can be prevented with careful maintenance and strict adherence to protocols.

The steps of processing

The processing cycle has four main stages, regardless of whether the processing is automatic or manual. The aim of the cycle is to produce a radiograph with a diagnostic image that can be immediately viewed and stored for future reference (Figure 9.1).

The four stages are:

- Development
- Fixing
- Washing
- Drying

Development

This is the first stage. During this stage, the latent image is converted into a visible image. During development the silver halide grains are reduced to metallic silver while the grains in the emulsion unaffected by the exposure do not change. This occurs through chemical reduction. The developer donates electrons to the silver ions in the silver halide, converting them to atoms of metallic silver. The sensitivity speck formed during exposure allows electrons from the developer to penetrate the grain and reduce the silver ions to metallic silver. If the film spends too long in the developer solution the developer may be able to penetrate unexposed grains causing chemical fogging to the resultant film.

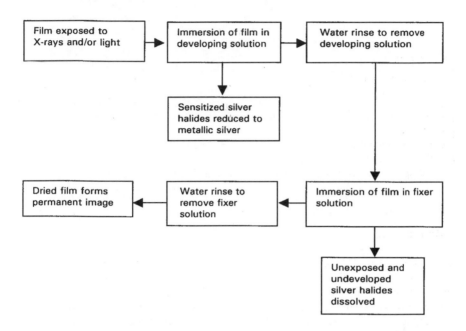

Figure 9.1. The processing cycle.

Fixing

This stage in the process will stop further development from occurring. This is achieved by ensuring that the solution is acidic, therefore providing a solution that will not allow the developing agents to work. Fixer will clear the image by removing silver halide crystals from the emulsion (Figure 9.2). The exposed crystals of silver halide have been converted to metallic silver, but the unexposed crystals remain. Unexposed silver halide grains account for about 60% of the total number of grains in the emulsion. These crystals will still be photosensitive and will darken as time goes by. This darkening will spoil the image. During fixing these silver halide crystals are converted to a compound that is soluble in water, allowing them to dissolve out of the emulsion. The time taken for this to occur is known as the clearing time.

In the final stages, fixing will prevent any further reactions from occurring to the film emulsion and ensure that the film emulsion hardens. The fixer hardens the gelatine, ensuring that it does not absorb too much water. This will in turn reduce the drying time necessary. Hardening will ensure that the emulsion is protected from damage during the washing and drying process, and during the viewing and storage of the film.

(a)   (b)   (c)

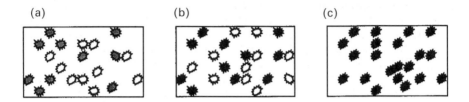

Figure 9.2. The effect of processing on the X-ray film emulsion. (a) Diagram showing silver halide grains in the film; grey areas are the latent image formed by exposure. (b) During development, metallic silver (black) is produced in the exposed grains. (c) During fixing, the silver halide grains are removed.

Clearing time	The time taken for a film to lose its milky appearance (image becomes transparent)
Fixing time	1.3 × clearing time

Washing

Washing is essential to prevent the continuing action of the chemicals used during both developing and processing.

In manual processing a wash tank is necessary between the developing and fixing stages. This will dilute the developer so that it will stop working and will also prevent contamination of the fixer.

During any form of processing a final wash is necessary. If the residue substances from development and fixing are not removed the film will gradually develop a yellow-brown (sepia) stain during storage. Dissolved salts may also crystallize on the surface of the film during storage if the film is not adequately washed.

The wash stage will only be effective if the amount of contamination in the water is lower than that in the emulsion. For this reason it is essential that running, fresh water is used.

The efficiency of the washing process will be affected by the amount of contaminant in the emulsion, the condition of the fixer, the flow and amount of water movement, the temperature of the water and the time taken to wash the film.

In automatic processing this time is usually about 10–20 seconds; in manual processing a minimum of 10 minutes is essential.

If the film is left in water for too long the emulsion may separate from the base, so careful monitoring is necessary.

Drying

During the drying process all of the surface water and most of the water from the emulsion must be removed. The drying time will depend on a number of factors including the wetness of the emulsion and the drying conditions (humidity, temperature and air circulation). If the drying temperature is too high, the film will become brittle. In automatic processing a squeegee will remove the surface water and evaporation will remove the water from the emulsion. This takes approximately 25 seconds. If the films are being manually dried, the films can be placed on a washing line in a dust-free environment or in a hot air cabinet. The temperature should meet the manufacturer's requirements.

Developer solution

Developing agents

The active agents in developer are hydroquinone and phenidone, and are used in combination depending on the manufacturer's requirements. Both reduce exposed silver bromide crystals to metallic silver by the donation of electrons. No developer is completely selective, so the agents that reduce exposed crystals the quickest are used. These agents have a strong smell, and can cause staining to clothing and dermatitis if they are in contact for any period of time. When the two compounds are used together the oxidation of hydroquinone will kick start the phenidone. This is known as super-additivity.

Preservative

This will slow the deterioration of the developer by producing an inert (unreactive) sulphonate that will slow the oxidation of the developer that usually occurs over time. The preservative is usually potassium metabisulphate.

Accelerator

This will maintain the alkalinity of the developer solution at about a pH of 9.6–10 (neutral is pH 7). An alkali solution will increase the rate of chemical reaction and maintenance of the pH at these levels will give adequate speed while still controlling the activity of the developer. The compound used is usually either sodium or potassium hydroxide.

Restrainer

This will improve the selectivity of the developer, reducing the levels of chemical fogging. The development process produces potassium bromide, which is a good restrainer, or a more powerful restrainer (benzotriazole) can be added in the manufacture process.

Sequestering agents

These are added to the developer to prevent the build up of a calcium sludge that may effect the processing of the film. This is usually EDTA (ethylene diamine-tetra-acetic acid) or a sodium salt.

Solvent

The solvent in developer is water. This dissolves the developer chemicals and all the processing by-products. The water will also make the emulsion layer swell allowing the developing agents to penetrate the emulsion and reach the silver halide crystals more easily.

Other additions

Hardener reduces the emulsion swelling and softens the emulsion. A wetting agent reduces the surface tension of the developer and will also prevent frothing of the surface. A fungicide will also prevent or reduce fungal growth.

S	Solvent
O	Other additive
A	Accelerator
P	Preservatives
R	Restrainer
A	A buffer
D	Developing agents
S	Sequestering agent

Fixer

The use of a fixer will give a permanent image and stop development. The fixer solution must be able to convert unexposed silver bromide into a form that can be washed off. This is known as conversion. It must have no effect on exposed crystals.

Fixing agent

This agent will diffuse into the emulsion and will react with the silver halides. This will produce silver sulphate, ammonium bromide and ammonium argento-thiosulphate. The compound used is ammonium thiosulphate as it is cheap and easy to prepare. It will also penetrate into the film quickly, reducing the chances of the film fogging. The ammonium thiosulphate will change the unexposed areas of the film from a milky white to a transparent appearance.

Solvent

The solvent used is water. This has a neutral pH and is cheap as well as readily available. This will dissolve into the emulsion carrying with it the dissolved fixer chemicals.

Acidifier

The acidifier will stop development preventing dichroic fog. This is seen as a green/blue-tinged stain when the image is viewed in reflective light and a pink stain when viewed with transmitted light. The deposit of very fine silver particles causes this over the surface of the film. The acidifier will neutralize the alkali developer.

   The acidifier will also allow the hardener to work. This is pH dependent and so acetic acid with a pH of 4–4.5 is used.

Buffer

This will maintain the pH of the fixer solution to within 0.2. Sodium acetate is usually used.

Preservative

This prevents decomposition of the fixer. As the ammonium thiosulphate breaks down sulphur is formed that will stop the fixer from working. The preservative is usually sodium sulphite, which is pH dependent.

Hardener

This will prevent damage to the film and allows drying. It is composed of an aluminium salt that will prevent the emulsion from swelling excessively. It will also prevent the emulsion from softening in the wash water or during the drying process.

Anti-sludging agent

The hardener will produce insoluble compounds that will form sludge on the bottom of the tank. Boric acid is used to reduce and prevent the formation of this sludge layer.

P	Preservative
A	Acidifier
F	Fixing agent
B	Buffer
A	Anti-sludging agent
S	Solvent
H	Hardener

Control of Substances Hazardous to Health Regulations (COSHH)

The chemicals involved in the developing of X-ray films are hazardous if inhaled or splashed on the skin. Great care should be taken when replenishing the tanks and during cleaning. Masks and gloves should always be worn, and there should be adequate ventilation at all times in the room surrounding the processor. Allergies can develop over time if there is unregulated exposure to the fumes given off by the chemicals.

Revision points

- There are four main stages to processing – development, fixing, washing and drying
- Development converts the latent image to a visible image
- Exposed silver halides are reduced to metallic silver
- Sensitivity speck allows developer solution to penetrate the grain
- Fixer stops the development process
- Fixer is acidic
- Fixer will clear the image by removing silver halide crystals from the emulsion
- Inadequate fixing will result in the silver halide grain changing colour with time a causing deterioration of the image
- The clearing time is the time taken for the film to lose its milky appearance
- Fixing time is 1.3 × clearing
- Washing is essential to prevent the continuing action of the chemicals
- Washing occurs between development and fixing in manual processing and after fixing in any type of processing
- Fresh running water must be used
- Drying removes surface water from the film and any residue water in the emulsion
- The developing agents are alkali
- Hydroquinone and phenidone are used as developing agents
- Preservative slows the oxidation of the developing agents
- An accelerator maintains the alkalinity of the solution
- A restrainer will improve the selectivity of the developer
- Sequestering agents reduce the build up of sludge in the tanks
- Ammonium thiosulphate is used as a fixing agent
- A solvent is used to dissolve the fixing agents. This is usually water
- An acidifier will stop the developer from working and prevent dichroic fog
- A hardener will prevent damage to the film and allow drying
- Preservative prevents decomposition of the fixer, buffers maintain the pH and an anti-sludge agent will stop the build up of sludge

---

Revision questions

1. Give the four main stages of processing in order
2. Describe what happens to the exposed silver halide crystals during development
3. How does the sensitivity speck assist in the development process?
4. Why is fixer solution acidic?
5. How are silver halide crystals removed from the emulsion?
6. Define clearing time and fixing time
7. What factors will affect the efficiency of the washing process?
8. What will happen if a film is left overnight in the wash tanks?
9. What happened during the drying process?
10. Name the two compounds in developing solution
11. How does the preservative in developer work?
12. Which part of the developing solution will prevent or reduce fogging of the film?
13. Why is water used as the solvent in fixer solution?
14. What is dichroic fog?
15. What are the two 'words' used to assist in remembering the components of fixer and developer solutions?

10 The production of a visible image

Objectives

• Manual processing
• Parts of the automatic processor
• Replenishment
• Silver recovery
• The darkroom
• Other methods of processing
• Viewing the radiograph

Introduction

The processing of a radiograph is dependent on suitable equipment, and the safe and efficient use of this equipment. The chemistry involved is common to both manual and automatic processing, and a basic understanding of the function of the chemistry involved will assist in development of accurate and effective processing skills.

Manual processing

Manual processing is the process of developing an exposed film when no automatic machine is available. This method of developing films involves the manual immersion of films in separate tanks. This method of processing is time consuming, and will take a longer period of time to produce a dry radiograph ready for viewing and storage.

Specific equipment should be available for this process:

Manual processing unit or trays
Hangers for suspending the films
A drying cabinet
Stirring rods for the fixer and developer
Accurate timer
A thermometer to clip onto the edges of tanks or floating
Protective masks and gloves
Clean, running water

Tanks

The films are processed in either deep narrow tanks or shallow trays. There should be separate trays for the developer, rinse, fixer and wash. In a veterinary practice the trays may be cat litter trays used solely for the developing process. Whatever type of tank is used, it should be capable of holding at least one 35–43 cm film totally immersed.

Deep tanks are usually made from stainless steel or chemical resistant plastics. The types in use usually have a 5-gallon capacity. The tanks should be covered at all times to decrease the oxidation of the developer. Covering the tanks will also prevent evaporation of the solutions and the entry of dust and animal hairs.

The tanks should be cleaned regularly at least when the chemistry is changed. This should involve emptying the tank completely and scrubbing all the sides of the tank and cleaning with fresh water.

Temperature

The temperature of the solutions must be maintained to ensure that the chemicals are working at the optimum temperature. This is usually at about 20°C, but will depend on the manufacturers' guidelines. The tanks can be heated by a water jacket surrounding the tanks or an immersion heater. The use of a water jacket is more suitable for this type of processing as it can be accurately controlled and the chemistry is not directly heated. Direct heating can increase oxidation and will shorten the life of the chemistry. Algae can build up in the water jacket and so careful maintenance should be employed. The water jacket and wash tanks should be emptied and cleaned regularly and left empty when not in use. Regular cleaning of the tanks will prevent algae causing an artefact on the resultant image. Algae will attack the gelatine in the emulsion and have detrimental effects on image quality.

Film hangers

All films should be placed in hangers during development to reducing artefacts from handling and contamination. There are two types of hangers; channel hangers and spring clips.

Channel hangers are easy to use as the film slides into a channel top and bottom. These are however difficult to keep clean, as the chemicals will collect and dry in the bottom of the channels. This can lead to artefacts on the films.

Spring clip hangers are harder to use at first and can scratch other films in the tanks, but they are easy to care for and keep clean.

Protocol for manual processing

1. Check the levels and temperature of the chemistry, make up as required and mix thoroughly
2. Turn off all white lights and ensure that the safelights are on. Lock the door to the room
3. Unload the cassette and place the film in a hanger

4. Place the film in the developer and ensure that the developer coats the emulsion evenly and completely
5. Start the clock and leave the film in the developer for the recommended time – do not remove the film before the recommended time (usually 4 min)
6. Place the film in the rinse tank a couple of times to stop the developer from working and wash some of the chemical off
7. Place the film in the fix tank and leave it for a minimum of 8 min
8. Remove the film from the fixer and place it in running water for a minimum of 30 min
9. Hang the film to dry
10. Reload the cassette ready for use

Parts of the automatic processor

Automatic processing works on the same principle as manual processing except that it is carried out by a machine with a series of rollers and the dry to dry time is usually much quicker than with manual processing. The automatic processor is usually simple to operate and maintain (see Figure 10.1).

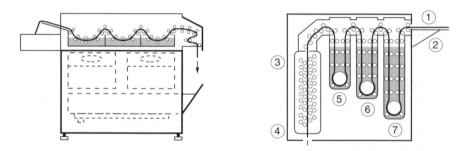

Figure 10.1. Horizontal and vertical automatic processors. 1, Film entry; 2, feed tray; 3, dryer; 4, film exit; 5, wash; 6, fixer; 7, developer.

Film transport system

The film is initially taken into the processor through a film feed system. This will contain a microswitch that detects the film and will calculate the correct amount of replenishment required. The microswitch will also detect when the film is totally in the processor and indicate that another film can be entered or the white light can be switched back on. The film is carried through the tanks through a series of rollers. These will press the solution onto the surface of the film and will also squeegee excess chemistry off the surface of the film as it leaves the tanks. To alter the amount of time the film spends in each tank, the depth of the tank is altered, rather than having a complicated gear system. The transportation may either be vertically through a series of deep tanks or horizontally through a series of shallow trays.

Water systems and drainage

Water within the processor will assist in the control of temperature. If the water is not switched on with the processor, the developer and fixer solutions will overheat and will not work effectively. The temperature used in automatic processors is usually higher than that for manual processing. The water for washing is usually cold although slightly warm water is more efficient. To prevent the formation of algae the water is on timer control so that it is constantly changed and moved through the system.

   The drainage of water and other products from the processor are controlled by the 'Deposit of Poisonous Waste Act 1972' and these must be adhered to carefully. The developer and fixer solutions should not enter the public sewer without the consent of the local authority and if possible the waste fixer and developer should be stored and disposed of separately through a recognized company who deal in waste chemicals.

Dryer systems

The film is dried using hot air at 50–60°C. The air is warmed either by an electric heater or infrared lamps surrounded by air blowers. On entry into the dryer more rollers squeegee the film so the water to be removed from the film is minimal.

Care of the automatic processor

The automatic processor needs as much care and cleaning as a manual processor if not more. The tanks and rollers must be cleaned regularly (once a week) to stop build-up of the residual chemicals that may impair the function of the processor. The build-up of residual chemicals will speed up the deterioration of the remaining chemicals, may cause scratches to the film and may cause the film to override the rollers. Details of cleaning and maintenance regimes are usually supplied with the processor.

Replenishment

Replenishment is an essential part of the maintenance of the processor whether it is manual or automatic. General radiography will result in about 40% of the silver on the film being used. The remainder will be washed out into the developer and fixer solution along with the by-products of the processing cycle, leading to a reduction in the concentration of the developer and fixer. The amount of replenishment will depend on the throughput of X-rays. As throughput increases the amount of replenishment for each film will decrease, as there is less time for the solutions to degenerate. If a thicker emulsion is used, then more chemicals will be carried over from one tank to another and the amount of replenishment for each film will need to be increased.

Replenishment during manual processing

Replenishment is not easy with manual processing and the levels of chemistry in the respective tanks should be monitored and topped up. The average life of developer is about 10 weeks, regardless of the amount of use. Even without any use the condition of the developer will deteriorate.

If the throughput is low it may be more economical to dish develop films and only make up 1-gallon containers of fixer and developer. This can then be decanted into litter trays or other similar containers when required. The fixer and developer can then be discarded after use. The pre-made containers of fixer and developer can be stored at room temperature out of direct sunlight until they are needed.

Replenishment in an automatic processor

Every time a film is fed into the processor the entry roller system will trigger the replenishment system. This will allow replenisher solution to be pumped into the tanks in the processor. The new solution is mixed with the old by the action of the rollers, and excess drains out through an overflow into the silver recovery unit and the drainage system. The replenishment chemicals are held in reservoir tanks or in smaller units in plastic containers. Maximum efficiency can be obtained through the use of an automixer. This is a unit that will automatically mix the fresh chemistry and store it until it is required by the processor. This is much cleaner and saves time when compared to manual mixing. It will also ensure accurate and total mixing of the chemicals and water.

Starter solution and mixing chemicals

When the processor is started from dry a starter solution containing potassium bromide and acetic acid is needed. This will depress the pH of the developer, decreasing the activity of the solution. This will control the activity of the developing agents and increase the selectivity of the new developer solution.

Developer is usually supplied in two or three containers containing the main constituents that are mixed with water.

Fixer comes in two separate containers. Part A contains the replenisher with most of the chemicals and Part B contains the hardener. This hardener can cause burns and allergies if it is inhaled. If Parts A and B are stored together they will deteriorate and should only be put in the same container when they are required for use.

Silver recovery

Silver can be recovered from either used fixer solution or from old discarded films. The films and fixer solution can be collected and recycled by a firm that specializes in refining silver. If the radiographic throughput of the veterinary practice is constant the cost of removing the films and used fixer solution will be compensated by the amount of silver recovered. Once the silver recovery has taken place, depending on the methods used, the fixer solution can be re-used. Approximately 98% of the total silver in fixer solution can be reclaimed. This can be carried out using electrolysis or the depositing of silver on a steel wool column.

As the sources of silver become scarcer, recovery of used silver in this form is essential to reduce the cost of industrial silver and maintain silver for future generations.

The darkroom

The darkroom is the room where films are processed or placed into the automatic processor and the area in which cassettes will be reloaded. It will also provide a safe area for the handling of films. The room should be easily accessible to all. It should not be near any damp or hot areas with good ventilation and must have a reliable source of electricity and water. The room must be away from any sources of direct or scattered radiation.

If manual processing is taking place the darkroom should have distinct wet and dry areas so that contamination of films and screens does not take place. The dry area (present in both manual and automatic processing environments) should have a workbench where cassettes can be open and closed easily. The bench should be made of wood or linoleum so that static build up is avoided. Film storage should be available in the dry area either in the form of a hopper or light tight drawers. Boxes of films should not be stored on the work surfaces.

The wet area should contain the manual processor or tanks and the drying area. This should be separate from the dry area (see Figure 10.2).

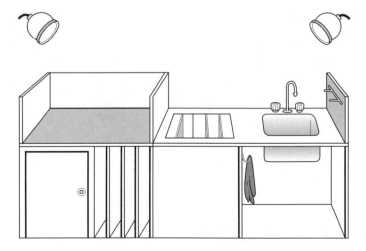

Figure 10.2. Layout of a darkroom with dry and wet areas.

Size

The room should have a minimum floor space of $10 \, m^2$. This will provide adequate room to move around and safely use the manual processing tanks and film hoppers or drawers storing the films.

Floors

The floor should be light coloured composed of a non-porous, non-slip material that can be easily cleaned and maintained. As the environment is usually poorly lit, then trip hazards should not be present and obstacles should be kept to a minimum.

Walls and ceilings

The walls should be light to reflect as much safelight as possible into the room and onto the working surfaces. This may reduce the number of light fittings required to give a suitable intensity of light to work with. The walls should be easy to keep clean and in wet processing areas they should be tiled for easy maintenance and cleaning.

Ceilings should be white or cream and a paint that could flake (emulsion) should be avoided.

Ventilation

The room should be well ventilated to provide a safe and comfortable environment for staff. The area should not be too hot or humid as this could damage the films stored in the room.

Doors

Where a single door is used care must be taken to ensure accidental entry during processing is avoided. The door should be light sealed and have a lock or some description. If there is space a double-door system is ideal. This involves two doors that will provide a light lock. The walls should be painted black to prevent the reflection of light into the dark room. If the room has windows there should be black light proof blinds provided that run in channels to prevent the light penetrating round the edges of the blinds (see Figure 10.3).

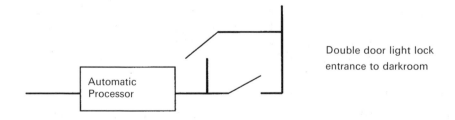

Double door light lock
entrance to darkroom

Automatic
Processor

Figure 10.3. Plan of a darkroom with a double door light lock entrance.

White lights

White lights are needed in the darkroom to allow safe and thorough cleaning of the floor and work surfaces. The white light is also needed for the safe maintenance and cleaning of the processor and any other equipment needed in the dark room. The lights should not be fluorescent as these give an afterglow that could cause fogging. Two switches should be provided. A light switch is needed near the door with a second switch nearer to the work surfaces. The switches should be away from the safelight switches or marked in some easily distinguishable way.

Safelights

A safelight is essential to prevent light affecting the film and causing fogging. All radiographic film is sensitive to white light and so the light must be filtered. A safelight is a box containing a low wattage (maximum of 25 W pearl light bulb) and a filter to remove the parts of the spectrum that the film is most sensitive to. The filter is a layer of gelatine, dyed to the appropriate colour between two sheets of glass. Most radiographic film is sensitive to green or blue light and so selecting a filter that will remove this light will result in reduced fogging of the film (see Figure 10.4).

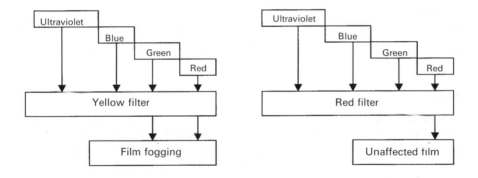

Figure 10.4. The effect of safelight colour on light transmission.

Even with the use of suitable safelights, fogging to the film will occur and the efficiency of the safelights should be monitored. If a safelight becomes cracked it will causing fogging to the radiographs. Handling of films under safelight conditions should be kept to a minimum, as fogging and a loss of contrast will eventually be seen on all films.

Indirect safelighting

This type of safelight will give general illumination to the darkroom. The light is directed towards the ceiling and is then reflected back into the room. The safelight will usually have filters above and below providing direct and indirect illumination. These should be at least 2.1 m above the floor of the darkroom (see Figure 10.5(a)).

Direct safelights

This is usually in the form of a beehive safelight. This will direct the light straight onto the work surface and the film. This type of safelight should be at least 1.2 m from the work surface. This type of safelight is the most suitable type of light for area in which cassettes are loaded and unloaded (see Figure 10.5(b)).

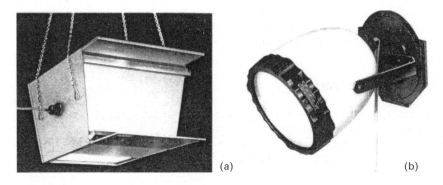

(a)   (b)

Figure 10.5. (a) Indirect (hanging) safelight and (b) direct (beehive) safelight.

Other methods of processing

The effect of X-rays can be demonstrated on media other than conventional radiographic film. This is a good solution if processing facilities are not available especially during theatre cases using fluoroscopy or when working in remote locations away from conventional processing facilities.

Polaroid

Polaroid imaging uses a special type of film that works in reverse to conventional radiographic film. The Polaroid film usually comes in a pack with negative and positive films and a pod of jellified processing chemicals. The film is exposed in the usual way and then placed into a custom-made processor. This will use a series of rollers to break the pod of chemicals and spread it evenly over the film. The latent image is formed in the silver halide of the negative sheet. During processing the jellified chemicals will develop both exposed and unexposed silver halides in the negative emulsion. Areas on the negative that have received an exposure will have black silver deposited; the unexposed areas will donate silver ions to the crystalline silver layer on the positive film. This is the image that will be viewed. It will be the reverse to the negative image.

Thermal imaging

The image is produced by heat. Light produces a latent image on special heat sensitive paper and then it is developed using heat. This dries the silver in the paper to form the image. Thermal imaging can be used to print a radiographic image from a television monitor. This is of use during fluoroscopic examinations where no other means of image storage or retrieval (10 cm film or video) is available.

Video

Video images can be used to store a real-time image (as it happens) during fluoroscopy. This gives the option to view the procedure repeatedly and actually requires a lower patient dose. The main disadvantage of this method is a reduction in image resolution.

Viewing the radiograph

The methods employed to view a radiograph can greatly improve (or destroy) the quality of an image. A viewing box contains fluorescent tubes with a reflective back. The box has a Perspex front that provides an even density across the whole screen. The most desirable features of a viewing box are:

- Light of an even intensity from edge to edge
- Light as white as possible
- Minimal heat given off from the light source
- Facility to vary brightness
- High intensity spot (bright light)
- Transparent film grips

The box should be regularly cleaned inside and out. This will prevent a build up of dust that will affect the intensity of the light provided. The Perspex should be cleaned using an antistatic polish.

Revision points

- Manual and automatic processing follow the same basic principles
- Manual processing relies on the use of tanks and the immersion of films in the solution by hand
- The temperature of the solution is maintained through the use of a water jacket or immersion heater
- All films for manual development need to be placed in film hangers
- Automatic processors rely on a film transportation system to take the film from one tank to the next
- Squeegee rollers remove excess chemistry between tanks
- The time the film spends in each tank is altered by the depth of the tank
- Water is used to maintain the temperature of an automatic processor
- Algae should not be allowed to build up in the wash tanks as it will cause artefacts on the radiographic image
- Films are dried using an electric heater or infrared lamps surrounded by blowers
- Waste products should be disposed of following the guidelines set out in the 'Deposit of Poisonous Waste Act 1972'
- Regular cleaning and maintenance should be carried out on all processors
- Replenishment will replace used and tired chemistry each time a new film is placed into the processor
- Replenishment will maintain the concentration and activity of the active agents without the need to dispose of all of the solution
- Developer solution should be changed every 10 weeks regardless of the amount of use it has had
- Starter solution is needed when fresh developer solution is brought into use
- Silver recovery should be utilized where possible for economic and ecological reasons
- The darkroom should be a room used solely for the processing of films
- It should be light tight with reflective walls, floor and ceilings to utilize the available safelight
- Doors should be designed to prevent accidental opening
- The room should be well ventilated, not too hot or humid
- Safelights are essential to prevent the fogging of films
- The maximum light source should be a 25 W pearl light bulb
- A red filter should be used
- The colour of safelight should be selected to eliminate the colours of light that the film is sensitized to
- Handling of film under a safelight should be kept to a minimum to prevent fogging
- Safelights can be direct or indirect
- Images can be stored through thermal imaging, Polaroid images and development or the use of a video
- The radiograph should be viewed on a suitable custom-made viewing box
- This provides an even density of light that is as close to white as possible

Revision questions

1. *List five pieces of equipment necessary for manual processing*
2. *How should manual processing tanks be maintained?*
3. *How is the temperature controlled during manual processing?*
4. *Describe two types of film hanger*
5. *How does the film transport system of an automatic processor work?*
6. *Give two uses for water in an automatic processor*
7. *How can fixer and developer solution be disposed of once it is used if suitable drainage is not available?*
8. *Describe the daily care needed to maintain an automatic processor*
9. *How does replenishment in an automatic processor work?*
10. *What is starter solution and how should it be used?*
11. *Describe the problems encountered when mixing and storing fixer solution*
12. *Where can silver be recovered?*
13. *If you were designing a darkroom what factors in the design would be important?*
14. *How does a safelight work?*
15. *List four of the most desirable features of a viewing box*

Control of the primary beam and scatter

11

Introduction

Control of the primary beam is important in the maintenance of high radiation safety standards. If the primary beam is not limited, there will be increased levels of scattered radiation produced leading to an increased risk of exposure to the radiographer. Collimation in whatever form will also improve the visual quality of the resultant image.

Cones

This is a tapered metal structure made of steel or brass. The cone can be either cylindrical or truncated (Figure 11.1).

Truncated Cone   Cylindrical Cone

Figure 11.1. Cone shapes.

The cone is open at both end and is attached to the tube port. The cone does not allow the primary beam to be collimated to the object. The size of the field will depend on the focal spot to film distance, the length of the cone, the distance from the anode to the end of the cone and the overall diameter of the cone. All cones have a figure on the side. If the distance from the focal spot to the film is divided by this figure, the diameter of the field will be shown (see Figure 11.2).

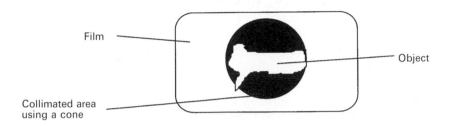

Figure 11.2. Schematic illustration of the effect of a cone on the primary beam.

Diaphragms

The diaphragm is a fixed piece of metal with a rectangular or circular aperture. This will limit the beam to an area, but must be used at a set focal film distance. At the set focal spot to film distance the size of the diaphragm will be limited to a predetermined size (see Figure 11.3).

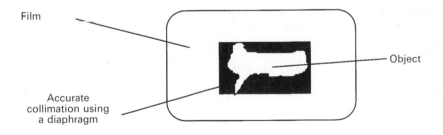

Figure 11.3. Schematic illustration of the effect of a diaphragm on the primary beam.

Radiation safety and the use of cones and diaphragms

The use of cones and diaphragms should be limited in practice as light beam diaphragms are now found on most machines. The purchase of replacement machines, without a light beam diaphragm or a moveable collimator should be avoided. The ionizing radiation guidelines do not prohibit their use, but limitation of the primary beam is not adequate using cones and diaphragms. This may reduce radiation safety through increased scattered radiation and increased use of the primary beam.

Light beam diaphragm

This is an aluminium box that is lead lined, fixed below the port on the tube. The bottom of the box has a Perspex window. Just above the Perspex window there are two pairs of adjustable lead leaves. The opposing faces are bevelled at 45° to give total closure (see Figure 11.4).

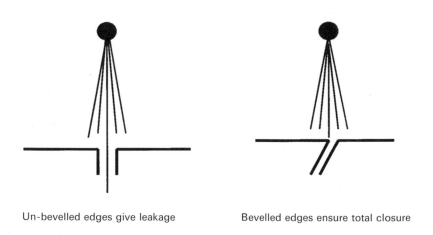

Un-bevelled edges give leakage   Bevelled edges ensure total closure

Figure 11.4. Effect of bevelled diaphragm leaves on the effectiveness of limitation of the primary beam.

A light is displayed at the same angle as the primary beam through the use of a series of mirrors. The mirror does not alter the beam. The unit has an automatic timer so that it will switch off after a set period of time, therefore preventing it from overheating. The diaphragm box should rotate to give flexibility on patient position and collimation.

Beam centring devices

These devices will allow control of the alignment of the tube to the patient and the area of irradiation to the patient. This is usually built in to the Perspex window on the bottom of the light beam diaphragm. The Perspex will have a cross marking the centre of the focal spot and light will demonstrate the edges of the collimated field. In older machines the centring device may need to be removed before the exposure is made as it may show on the radiograph.

Factors affecting scattered radiation

Secondary radiation is any radiation other than the primary beam. Any object that has been radiated can produce secondary radiation. If this secondary radiation is in any direction other than that of the primary beam it is known as scatter. This can also be in the form of backscatter from the table or the cassette.

Patient size

If the patient is large the overall volume of the patient will be greater and this will increase the amount of scatter generated. This can be reduced through the use of a compression band that will reduce the volume of tissue in any one place at a given time. This in turn will reduce the scatter produced and increase the contrast of the resultant image.

kV

The voltage selected for an examination will alter the amount of scatter produced. As the wavelength of the primary beam increases with an increase in kV, so the amount of scatter reaching the film will increase. The amount of Compton scatter will increase as the kV increases.

Function of grids

The grid has two functions:

- The grid will absorb secondary scattered radiation that may have a detrimental effect on the final image
- The grid will allow the primary beam to pass through unaffected to form the useful image on the film

Construction of a grid

The grid is usually seen as a sheet of metal from the outside, but the internal structure is made up of two very distinct parts; the lead strips and radiolucent spaces. The outside of the grid is made of aluminium as it is strong and gives high precision. The aluminium casing will also prevent moisture entering the grid and will give it rigidity (see Figure 11.5).

Lead strips

The lead strips will absorb the scattered radiation that does not pass through the radiolucent spacers. The lead will absorb the lower energy scattered radiation as it has a high atomic number and a high mass density. Lead is used, as it is cheap and fairly easy to shape. In any type of grid there will be a maximum of 40 strips of lead in every centimetre of grid.

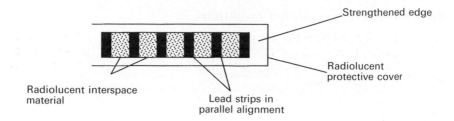

Strengthened edge

Radiolucent
protective cover

Radiolucent interspace
material

Lead strips in
parallel alignment

Figure 11.5. The construction of a parallel anti-scatter grid.

Radiolucent interspace

This is made of plastic, aluminium or carbon fibre. The material used must be rigid to maintain the position of the lead strips. The interspace will allow the primary beam to pass straight through whilst filtering the scattered radiation. Despite the primary beam passing straight through the interspace some of the primary beam will be absorbed by the lead strips and so a higher exposure will be necessary when using a grid (see Figure 11.6).

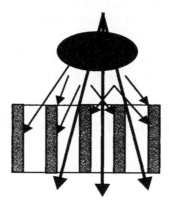

Figure 11.6. The effect of a grid on primary and secondary radiation.

Grid ratio

The grid ratio is the height of the strips to the width of the interspace. If the ratio is high, more scattered radiation will be absorbed. If a grid has a high ratio then a higher exposure must be used to compensate for the increase in absorption of the primary beam. Ratios range from 3:1 to 16:1 although the ratio in common use is 6:1

4:1	A ratio of 4:1 means that the heights of the lead strips are four times the width of the spacer
10:1	A ratio of 10:1 means that the heights of the lead strips are ten times the width of the spacer

Grid lattice

The grid lattice describes the lines per centimetre. This is the number of strips to each centimetre. As the number of lines increases so the exposure needed to produce a diagnostic radiograph increases but the amount of scatter absorbed also increases.

Grid factor

When a grid is used, the amount of exposure required also increases. The exposure factor increased is the mAs. The amount of exposure increase can be calculated. Depending on the type of grid used, the grid factor is usually about 4, but will depend on the grid factor.

Grid factor = exposure with the grid/exposure without the grid

Types of grid

Parallel

A parallel grid has lead strips that are vertical and parallel to each other. This type of grid is the most simple to use, as it does not have to be used with a specific focal film distance or specific centring point. The tube can be angled so long as it is parallel to the lead strips. This type of grid is also the cheapest to buy. Some cut-off of radiation will occur on the edges of the film because of the divergence of the primary beam (see Figure 11.7).

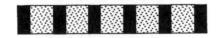

Figure 11.7. Parallel grid.

Focused

With this type of grid, the lead strips and interspacers are titled with an increasing angle further from the centre of the grid. This allows for the diverging primary beam on the edges of the useful beam to pass through the grid. If the lead strips were extended they would meet at a point in front of the grid. This is known as the grid focus and is where the tube should be positioned to get the maximum performance from the grid. Centring and focus to grid distance need to be accurate, otherwise cut off will occur. If the grid is used back to front cut off will occur (see Figure 11.8).

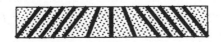

Figure 11.8. Focused grid.

Pseudo-focused grid

With this type of grid the lead slats are parallel, but tapered. This means that the diverging beam is able to pass through the grid without being absorbed, as it would be in a parallel grid (see Figure 11.9).

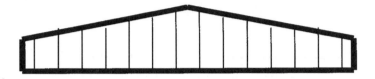

Figure 11.9. Pseudo-focused grid.

Cross-hatched parallel grid

This type of grid has parallel lead strips laid at 90° to each other. This gives excellent removal of scatter but does require a large increase in exposure. The positioning with this type of grid needs to be accurate (see Figure 11.10).

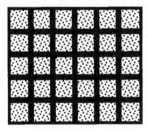

Figure 11.10. Cross-hatched parallel grid.

Moving grids (Potter–Bucky grid)

The use of a stationary grid will produce an image with very fine lines from the lead strips. To eliminate this effect the grid can be moved very rapidly to blur out the lines. This type of grid is usually parallel with the grid mounted beneath the tabletop. When the exposure is made the grid moves rapidly from side to side, on termination of the exposure the grid will stop moving. This movement must be smooth and uninterrupted (see Figure 11.11).

Choosing a grid

The choice of a grid will depend on the funds available at the time of choice and the type of work that it will be used for. A parallel grid is good for day-to-day veterinary work, but if funding allows, the use of a pseudo-focused grid would be the grid of choice. Cross-hatched parallel grids should be used if a large amount of farm animal or equine work is carried out.

A grid should be used when X-raying any patient or part of patient over 10 cm thick. Below this level scatter will not be of a level to influence the image quality.

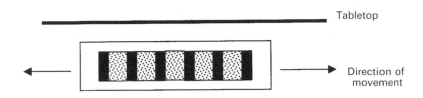

Figure 11.11. Moving grid (Potter–Bucky grid).

Problems with using a grid

Grids should be used with care otherwise a number of problems can be encountered. If a grid is dropped then bending of the lead strips is a possibility and this will have a detrimental effect on the function of the grid. The recommendations of the manufacturer should be followed at all time for the best results from the grid. This includes using the correct focal distance and using the grid the correct way round (grids have a back and a front) with the tube side facing the tube. If the grid is used back to front the primary beam will be absorbed on the edges and will only pass directly through in the middle of the film. This will give an image with cut-off, where the middle is adequately exposed, but the edges will have varying densities. This can also happen with incorrect centring or tilting of the grid or use of the wrong focus to grid distance.

Air-gap technique

If the exposure cannot be safely increased when using a grid with a large patient, then the air-gap technique can be used. This is an ideal technique for imaging the equine chest or spine. A gap is left between the patient and the film. The gap will allow the scatter produced in the body to be absorbed by the air due to the inverse square law. The scatter is of a lower energy. As the distance increases so the scatter will have a lower energy level and less of an effect on the film. The scattered radiation can also be lost through divergence after exiting the patient. The air gap should be a minimum of 15 cm up to a maximum of 300 cm (see Figure 11.12).

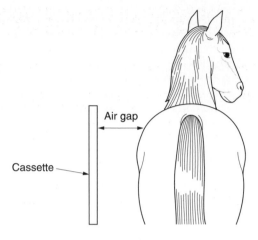

Figure 11.12. Air-gap technique.

Revision points

- Cones, diaphragms and collimators can limit the primary beam
- Radiation safety is improved by limiting the primary beam
- Cones fit onto the X-ray port and are either truncated or cylindrical
- Diaphragms are a fixed piece of metal with an aperture
- Light beam diaphragm collimators give most accurate limitation of the primary beam
- Light beam diaphragm has lead leaves with bevelled edges
- Scattered radiation is dependent on patient size and the kV used
- Grids absorb unwanted secondary radiation
- A grid is made up of lead strips spaced with a radiolucent material
- The lead strips absorb the scatter
- The grid ratio is the height of the strips to the width of the spaces
- Grids can be either parallel, focused, pseudo-focused or cross-hatched
- To eliminate grid lines the grid can be moved
- Care must be taken with grids to ensure that manufacturers' guidelines are followed
- The grid should be flat and in the correct orientation to the tube when used
- The air-gap technique can also remove scatter

Revision questions

1. Which of the following statements are incorrect when discussing collimation:
   (a) The area exposed should never be larger than the film size used
   (b) The useful beam should be limited to the smallest area practicable and consistent with the objectives of the examination
   (c) The beam should be collimated to the area of the largest cassette in general use
2. Give two ways of controlling the primary beam once it has left the X-ray tube
3. Why are the edges of the lead leaves in a collimator bevelled?
4. How does patient size affect the amount of scatter produced?
5. Describe the construction of a grid
6. What is the grid factor?
7. How are focused and pseudo-focused grids different?
8. What size of patient or patient part is suitable for using a grid to improve the image?
9. What is the air-gap technique?
10. What size should the air gap be as a minimum to be effective?

12 Radiographic image quality

Introduction

During the production of radiographs, a number of faults can occur, either human or mechanically generated. These can be detrimental to the diagnostic value of the radiograph. Through simple quality assurance and equipment care, these faults can be avoided, and if they do occur identification at an early stage can prevent unnecessary repeat radiographs and possible extended anaesthesia for the patient.

Sensitometry

Sensitometry is a way of assessing the performance of a film, screen, film/screen combination or a processor. To allow successful sensitometry, a sensitometry strip needs to be produced. This can be produced using a sensitometer. This is a device containing a controlled light source and filters. The combination of the light and filters will simulate the effect of light from the intensifying screens on a film. A step wedge can be used to provide a scale of graduated densities for sensitometry. A step wedge is a strip of aluminium with varying thickness of additional metal. Both the step wedge and sensitometer will produce an image with varying shades of grey. The exposure should always be made using the same machine or exposure factors. If these factors alter, then the density of the steps may alter, possibly leading to inaccurate analysis. The density of the film is assessed using a densitometer. This will compare the intensity of light incident on and transmitted through a selected area of film. This is known as the optical density. The details received through the use of the densitometer can be recorded and plotted. This will give a characteristic curve.

Sensitometry	Means of assessing film, screen or processor function
Sensitometer	A device used to produce a range of densities ready for analysis
Step wedge	Aluminium strips of increasing thickness exposed to produce a range of densities for analysis
Densitometer	Device used to assess the incident light falling on and transmitted through a radiographic film

Characteristic curve

The results obtained from the densitometer can be plotted to produce a characteristic curve (Figure 12.1). This is the log of the relative exposure against the density. The log of the relative exposure compresses the scale to give a suitable graph and ensures that two exposures will always have the same separation on the exposure scale. The relative exposure is obtained from the exposures used in the production of the step-wedge. From the graph the useful density of the film, the film latitude and exposure latitude can be calculated.

When the data are plotted the graph has three distinct areas, the shoulder, toe and straight-line portion. At the toe and shoulder, large variations in exposure factors result in very small changes in the optical density.

Toe

At the toe the levels of optical density are just above the base density and fog. In this region very small changes in density will result from changes in exposure factors. The toe is the area of under exposure on a diagnostic radiograph.

Straight-line portion

In the straight-line portion the image will be properly exposed and can be used to form a diagnostic image.

Shoulder

The shoulder is the area of the curve where further increases in exposure produce gradually smaller increases in density. This is the region of over exposure.

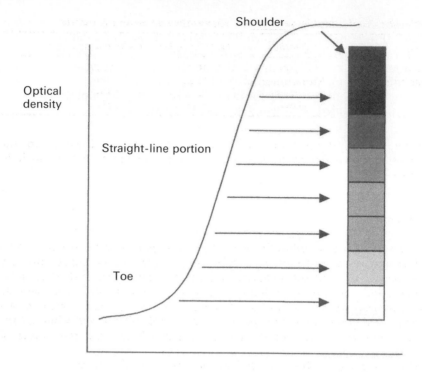

Figure 12.1. Characteristic curve of radiographic film.

Latitude

The latitude of a film describes the range of exposures that will ensure that a diagnostic image is possible. This can be determined from the characteristic curve. If a film has wide latitude there is a greater range of exposure factors that will produce a diagnostic image. If the film has narrow latitude, then the response of the film is more limited. Films with wide latitude will have a longer grey scale than films with narrow latitude. If the film has a high contrast, it will have narrow latitude (less grey range).

Density

The density of a film describes the amount of blackening on the resultant image. This subject density is related to the density of the part being examined. If a part of the patient is very dense and has a high atomic number, the number of X-ray photons passing through will be low. This results in a pale or clear area on the radiograph. If the area of interest is not dense and has a low atomic number such as air, the X-rays will pass through easily and will cause areas of blackness on the film (see Table 12.1).

Table 12.1. Radiographic density and appearance of different tissues

Tissue	Density	Atomic number	Appearance on X-ray
Bone	High	High	White
Water/muscle	Medium/high	High	Grey
Fat	Low/medium	Low	Grey
Air	Low	Low	Black

Photographic density may also be present due to fogging on the radiographic film due to storage conditions, processing conditions or light exposure.

Contrast

The term contrast describes the density between two adjacent structures on a radiographic image. If there is a wide range of grey on the image, but very little black and white, the image has a long scale of contrast. If there are a lot of black and white areas, but limited greys, on a radiographic image, then the image has a short scale of contrast. In diagnostic radiography a long contrast scale is ideal giving a wide range of grey but limited black and white on the image. Films that have a short scale of contrast will have a narrow range of latitude.

The contrast of a film is dependent on a number of factors:

- Tissue density and atomic number
- kV
- Object shape and thickness
- Film contrast
- Film fogging
- Use of contrast medium

All of these factors will alter the contrast of the image, although the degree each part plays is difficult to define.

Tissue density and atomic number

These two factors are closely related. An increase in atomic number and density will result in more X-ray photons being absorbed. If the tissue being radiographed is dense then a higher kV_p will be required. This will result in higher X-ray energy, and the presence of Compton scatter and the photoelectric effect. If the tissue has a lower density such as soft tissue and fat, then the kV_p required to penetrate the tissue will be lower.

kV

This is the most variable exposure factor when contrast is being determined. As the kV_p increases so the contrast scale increases. The use of a high kV_p will produce a wide range of grey scale (long scale of contrast). A low kV_p will produce an image with a lot of black and white, but a limited grey scale. The use of a low kV_p will need the use of higher mAs to produce an image of a similar density. This is not desirable, as it will increase the patient dose. An increased kV is used in chest radiography to 'flatten' the image and improve the contrast. In most situations the kV should be increased rather than time as movement blur with longer exposure times will reduce the image contrast.

Object shape and thickness

The shape and thickness of the body will alter the contrast of the radiographic image. If the area is very thin it will absorb less X-rays than an area with greater thickness. This can lead to uneven contrast across a radiograph and even through an organ if the thickness alters. This is seen in abdominal radiographs of deep-chested and thin dogs. The contrast is acceptable in one region (cranial or caudal), but the second area appears to be lacking in contrast due to a different thickness or absence of tissue. This can be overcome by placing lead shielding in the area of the primary beam in the caudal abdomen to fill in the area of missing tissue. This will increase the contrast of the caudal abdomen. The problem can also be overcome by taking two separate radiographs with different exposure factors to demonstrate the two areas.

Film contrast

The film contrast describes the latitude of a film. Films with a wide range of latitude will have a higher contrast giving a wider range of grey scale. This is due to the silver halide crystal shape or size in the film emulsion.

Film fogging

Film fogging is caused by poor storage of films or exposure to light or radiation including scattered radiation during the examination. Fogging will cause the film to have an overall greyness and a reduction in contrast.

Use of contrast medium

The contrast of an image can be improved through the use of contrast medium. All contrast media have high atomic numbers (iodine = 53, barium = 56) and this will absorb more X-ray photons. If the exposure factors are not altered to accommodate this absorption, then the contrast of the radiographic image will be enhanced. If negative contrast media (air) is introduced then exposure factors will need to be reduced to maintain the contrast on the radiographic image.

Contrast on a radiograph can be altered by:
Tissue density and atomic number
KV
Object shape and thickness
Film contrast
Film fogging
Use of contrast medium

Effects generated by the X-ray tube

The X-ray tube can generate artefacts that can be seen on the radiographic image. The three main artefacts are caused due to penumbra, focal spot size and the anode-heel effect.

Penumbra

Penumbra occurs due to the divergence of the primary beam. If a small focal spot (fine focus) is used then the X-ray beam will be formed in a very small area. This gives the latent image great detail, but increases the amount of heat received by one small area of the anode. Penumbra will give a slightly irregular or un-sharp image. This is more apparent in an image that has been produced using a double-sided emulsion and two intensifying screens. Penumbra may also occur with alteration of the collimation or alteration in the object film distance. By ensuring that the object is always as close to the film as possible, penumbra from distance can be reduced to a minimum (see Figure 12.2).

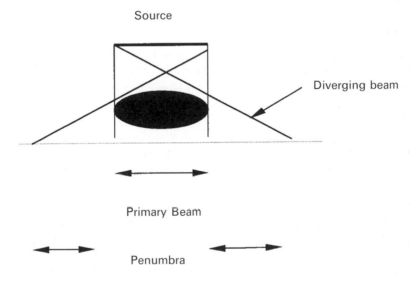

Figure 12.2. Demonstration of the areas covered by the primary beam and the diverging beam causing the penumbra effect.

Focal spot size

The focal spot is the area on the anode that the electrons strike. The focal spot is angled to decrease the area that it is possible for the electrons to strike. The smallest possible focal spot is achieved with a 7° angle, although the average is nearer to 20°. With a smaller focal spot, less divergence of the primary beam occurs, giving an image of a higher quality, as there is less distortion. The distortion would appear as very fine blurring or a reduction in the image quality. This will also reduce the amount of heat produced at the anode (see Figure 12.3).

Figure 12.3. The effect of focal spot size on the divergence of the primary beam.

The anode-heel effect

The anode-heel effect occurs due to the absorption of X-rays by the heel of the anode. This means that images on the cathode side of the radiograph will have a reduction in sharpness. There will also be some loss in sharpness seen on the anode side of the image, but this will be less noticeable. The heel effect increases with a reduction in anode angle and can cause a reduction in intensity of the beam by up to 45%.

Magnification

If the distance between the object being radiographed and the film is very large, magnification will occur. This is due to the primary beam continuing to diverge once it has passed through the object. This will distort the image and make it appear larger than it actually is. This can be used to our advantage in controlled situations where very small objects are being imaged using magnification. This is known as macro-radiography. The amount of magnification present can be calculated with a simple equation.

Magnification = focal film distance (FFD)/film object distance (FOD)

If it is essential to know how much magnification has occurred, such as fracture planning, a marker can be used. This marker will have a known length and can be imaged on the same film, next to the object. The magnification factor from this known size can then be applied to the object (see Figure 12.4).

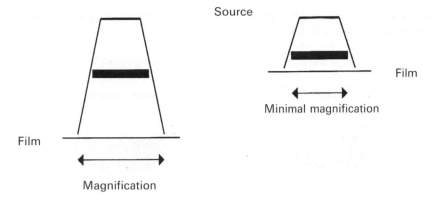

Source

Film

Minimal magnification

Film

Magnification

Figure 12.4. Changes in resultant image size with an increase in object film distance.

Distortion

This occurs if the object being imaged is not parallel to the primary beam. Distortion means that the object appears elongated or foreshortened. This can be detrimental to the image quality as size and shape of the object cannot be calculated accurately. This will also be seen at the periphery of the image and so care must be taken with interpretation of these areas (see Figure 12.5).

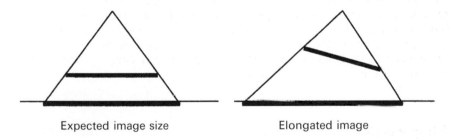

Expected image size   Elongated image

Figure 12.5. Effects of distortion on the length (or shape) of an object.

Distortion can be used to the radiographer's advantage to prevent superimposition of structures that may otherwise be on top of each other. This is especially the case in the skull examination.

Movement

Movement can have a detrimental effect on the image quality. It will result in the radiographic image being blurred with a reduction in overall contrast and possibly magnification if the movement has been away from the film. Movement of the patient can be reduced by using the shortest possible exposure time (with a high mA), ensuring that the tube support is stable and by using restraint. Restraint can be in the form of sedation or through the use of sandbags and ties.

Image quality can be affected by:

Density of the image
Contrast of the radiographic image
Penumbra
Focal spot size
Anode-heel effect
Magnification
Distortion
Movement

Altering exposure factors

Focal film distance (FFD)

The FFD is the distance from the focal spot of the X-ray tube to the film. This distance should be constant during all radiographic examinations if at all possible. If this distance is altered, the inverse square law can be applied. If the FFD is altered the number of electrons produced (and therefore X-rays) will need to be altered to produce a comparable radiograph. The mAs alterations can be calculated as below.

Old mAs $\times$ new distance^2/old distance^2 = new mAs

mAs

The mAs is the amperage applied to the tube multiplied by the time that it occurs over. In the ideal world the mA should be as high as possible with a short time. This will reduce movement blur from respiration or movement from the animal. It can be calculated as below. With rearrangement of the equation, changes in time or mA can be calculated.

mAs = mA $\times$ time (s)

kV

Alteration in the kV will alter the penetrating power of the primary beam. If the kV is higher, the mA can be reduced to give a radiograph of similar density. This does not mean, however, that the contrast will be similar. From a starting exposure, increasing the kV by 10 will require half the original mAs to give a radiograph of similar density.

60 kV	4 mAs	70 kV	2 mAs
80 kV	1 mAs	90 kV	0.5 mAs

Patient/part thickness

As the part being radiographed increases in size, so the kV will increase to allow adequate penetration. In practice with experience, this calculation will be carried out without measurements being necessary.

Use of grids

Grids reduce the amount of scattered radiation reaching the film, but in so doing, some primary beam or useful beam is absorbed. To compensate for this the exposure must be increased. The mAs should be multiplied by the grid factor.

Dressings

Wherever possible dressings should be removed; however, the following act as a guide:

Fibre glass/vet wrap and bandaging	$1.5 \times$ mAs
Plaster of Paris	$2 \times$ mAs
Wet plaster of Paris	$4 \times$ mAs

Exposure charts

These can be formed within a practice either as a daybook recording all examinations or built up over a period of time for different breeds of animal recorded by region of examination. To make the exposure chart an effective tool as many factors as possible need to be standardized. As a minimum this should be the FFD for each examination and the film/screen combination used. The chart can only be used as a guide because each animal and condition will require slightly different exposure factors. The exposure chart is specific to one particular machine, as all tubes will produce slightly different exposure factors, regardless of what is set.

Producing a high-quality radiograph

The production of a quality radiograph must take into account all of the factors described above. A satisfactory radiograph is said to be diagnostic.

A high-quality radiograph will provide sufficient views to make a diagnosis with adequate exposure factors and high-quality processing with no artefacts. The use of standard projections and accurate positioning with good collimation will assist in the production of a diagnostic radiograph.

To improve the quality of the radiographic image further, the animal must be free from any possible causes of artefacts. This includes dried mud, a wet coat or even spilt contrast medium if this has been administered to the animal previously. Collars, leads and dressings can also cause artefacts on the film and should be removed or moved away from the primary beam.

Commonly seen film faults

This description of film faults is not full but provides an outline of the more common film faults seen in veterinary radiography and solutions to help improve the image quality. Technique is the most common cause of film faults and this can be due to a number of very different reasons.

- Inadequate number of projections
- Lack of collimation
- No anatomical markers
- No patient identification or date
- Poor positioning or centring
- Movement
- Incorrect use of a grid
- Poor film screen contact
- Magnification
- Distortion
- Film/screen grainines

Appearance of film	Film fault	Reason for fault	Solution
Whole film too dark	Film over exposed	Incorrect settings	Decrease kV, mA or time
		Wrong focal-film distance	Increase focal-film distance
		Wrong film/screen combination	Use slower film/screen combination
Overall greyness to film	Film fogging	Film beyond expiry date	
		Poor film storage	Ensure correct storage conditions are maintained
		Film affected by scattered radiation	Ensure a grid is used and store cassettes away from radiation
		Film exposed to light	Check for stray leaks in the dark room and ensure that the safelight is correct
Overall greyness to film	Over development	Incorrect formula	Ensure chemistry is correctly diluted

Table (*continued*)

Appearance of film	Film fault	Reason for fault	Solution
		Developer overheated	Maintain correct temperature
		Film left in developer too long	Check immersion times carefully
		Developer contaminated with fixer	Make a fresh solution
Whole film too light	Film under exposed	Incorrect settings	Increase kV, mA or time
		Wrong focal-film distance	Decrease focal-film distance
		Wrong film/screen combination	Use faster film/screen combination
		Normal exposure used with a grid	
		Cassette used back to front	
Overall lightness to film	Under development	Developing time too short	Adjust developing time
		Developer below temperature	Maintain correct temperature
		Developer too dilute	Check mixing and dilution
		Developer exhausted	Make a fresh solution
Whole film clear	No exposure	Exposure not made correctly	
		Film placed in fixer before developer	
White areas	Bright white specks or object	Material between screen and film	Clean screens
	White area as a bright spot	Chemical spill on screen	Ensure cassettes are stored closed
	White splash marks on film	Fixer splashes on film before developing	Ensure strict darkroom practice
	Fingerprint	Fingers contaminated with fixer	Make sure that hands are clean and dry before handling films

Table (*continued*)

Appearance of film	Film fault	Reason for fault	Solution
Black areas	Straight clear strip at top of film	Developer tank levels are low	Check tank levels before processing
	Clear strip across middle of film	Scratches to emulsion of film through handling or poor processing	Handle films carefully and carryout regular cleaning of the processor
	Straight scratches or marks	Film dropped on floor or handled roughly during processing	
	Crescent marks on film	Pressure marks from finger nails	Handle film carefully
	Dots or tree pattern on film	Static electricity	Do not wear nylon Handle films carefully
	Splashes and streaks	Film splashed before processing with any liquid apart from fixer	Maintain carefully dark room procedures
	Black irregular border on all sides of the film	Light leakage from the edges of the cassette	Make sure cassettes are properly shut and are not damaged
	Black strip on end of film	Light leakage	Check film storage Do not lift lid off developer tanks during processing
			Allow film to enter automatic processor before using white light
	Linear black lines along full length of film	Pressure from rollers in processor	Keep rollers clean Check springs on roller assembly Do not pull films out of the dryer
Manual processing problems	Streaks and runs on films	Film hangers dirty	Routinely clean hangers to prevent the build up of chemicals
	Film dark at top with the lower half lighter	Uneven development	Always stir the developer before use
		Insufficient agitation	Move the films slightly once they are in the

Table (*continued*)

Appearance of film	Film fault	Reason for fault	Solution
	Film cloudy and streaky, possibly with a sticky surface	Insufficient fixing	Make sure the film has sufficient time in the fixer Change chemicals regularly
	Brown staining all over the film	Insufficient fixing	Make sure fixing time is adequate Change fixer regularly
	Uneven yellow or pale brown staining	Insufficient washing	Wash films for at least 30 minutes with fresh running water
	Grey speckles all over the exposed part of the film	Wash water stagnant and dirty	Keep tanks empty when not in use and clean regularly to prevent the build up of algae

---

Revision points

- Sensitometry assesses the performance of films, film/screen combinations or a processor
- A sensitometry strip is necessary for accurate assessment
- A step-wedge produces an image with varying densities
- A densitometer can be used to assess the incident light falling on and being transmitted through radiographic film
- Sensitometry results are recorded to form a characteristic curve
- The characteristic curve has three parts – shoulder, straight line and toe
- Latitude is the range of exposures that will ensure a diagnostic image on a radiographic film
- Density is the degree of blackening on a film
- The density of an image will depend on the atomic number of the part under investigation
- Contrast is the difference in density between two adjacent structures
- Contrast will depend on the patient density, kV selected, object shape and thickness, film contrast, film fogging, and the use of contrast medium
- Penumbra is caused by divergence of the primary beam
- A small focal spot size will reduce divergence, penumbra and blurring of the image
- The anode-heel effect may cause blurring of the image at the cathode end of the image
- Magnification will occur if the distance between the object and the film is large
- Distortion will occur if the object being imaged is not parallel with the primary beam
- Movement can cause blurring and reduction in sharpness of the film
- Changing the focal-film distance, mAs, kV, patient or part thickness, the use of a grid or the presence of dressings can alter exposure factors.
- Exposure charts need to be formulated for the machine in use
- Film faults will have a detrimental effect on image quality and can be eliminated by care and maintenance of equipment

Revision questions

1. What is the use of sensitometry and densitometry?
2. Describe how a sensitometric strip is produced and used
3. What are the two values used when plotting a characteristic curve?
4. Name the three parts of a characteristic curve
5. What is latitude?
6. How will bone, air, fat and water appear on a radiograph?
7. What does contrast describe?
8. If a film has a long scale of contrast, does it have wide or narrow latitude?
9. How will kV alter the contrast of a radiograph?
10. If negative contrast medium is being used, should the exposure factors be increased or decreased?
11. How does penumbra occur?
12. What is the anode-heel effect?
13. An increase in what factor will cause magnification?
14. What will distortion do to a radiographic image?
15. How can movement be avoided?
16. If the focal–film distance is altered, how can you calculate the change in mAs necessary to produce a similar image?
17. If the kV increases by 10, what will happen to the mAs
18. What changes in exposure factors will a dressing of wet plaster of Paris require to give a diagnostic radiograph?
19. How can an over developed film be corrected on the repeat processing?
20. What type of film fault will produce bright white specks on the radiograph?

13 Alternative imaging techniques

Objectives

Tomography
Fluoroscopy
Digital imaging
Computerized tomography (CT)
Magnetic resonance imaging (MRI)
Ultrasound
Nuclear scintigraphy

Introduction

In veterinary practice, the imaging modalities available are limited, but an understanding of all the available possibilities and how these would benefit a patient is essential. Conventional radiography can be expanded to include tomography and fluoroscopy. Ultrasound is becoming more available to practices as the price of equipment falls and more freelance imaging services become available. An understanding of the possibilities and the limitations of ultrasound, magnetic resonance imaging (MRI), computerized tomography (CT) and nuclear scintigraphy will benefit the care and treatment of a patient.

Tomography

The use of tomography is limited in smaller practice settings, but an understanding of the principles will improve understanding of the way in which CT works.

Tomography allows the size, depth, position and shape of organs to be shown. The film and X-ray tube are co-ordinated to move about a fixed point known as the fulcrum. All structures lying along the same level as the fulcrum will be demonstrated as a sharp image. Anything above or below this level will be blurred. As the angle of the tube movement increases, so the thickness of the sharp image layer decreases (see Figure 13.1).

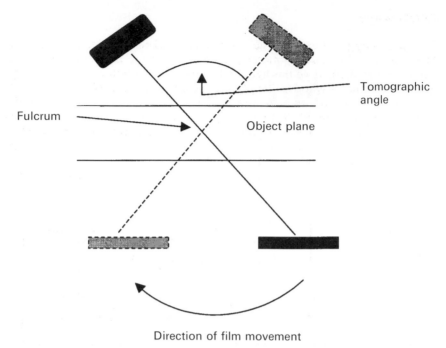

Tomographic angle

Fulcrum

Object plane

Direction of film movement

Figure 13.1. Movement of tube and film during a tomogram.

Uses of tomography

Examples of the use of tomography are the demonstration of kidney poles during intravenous urography or the demonstration of the mandible using panoramic tomography (Figure 13.2).

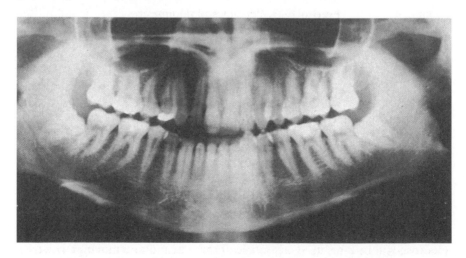

Figure 13.2. Human panoramic tomogram of the mandible.

Fluoroscopy

The fluoroscopy unit uses a basic X-ray tube attached to an image intensifier. This converts the X-rays emerging from the patient into light, and then multiplies the intensity of this light and converts it to photoelectrons through the use of a photocathode. The photocathode directs the electrons towards the output phosphor and an anode. The photoelectrons arriving at the output phosphor are 50–70 times brighter. This reduces the dose which is necessary to produce a suitable image. The photoelectrons are then used to form a television image that can be viewed. The quality of the image obtained is only as good as the monitor displaying the image. The size of the focal spot can be altered to magnify the image and enhance viewing further (see Figure 13.3).

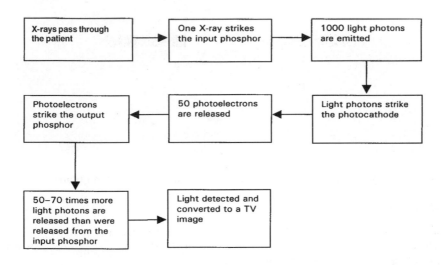

Figure 13.3. Principles of fluoroscopy.

The image displayed on the monitor will appear as the reverse of a conventional radiograph. Bone will be shown as black and the lungs will appear as white. The image produced using fluoroscopy, gives a moving image that can be recorded on video or it can be stored on 10 cm × 10 cm film in the normal way. These films are exposed using a very short exposure time so that multiple exposures can be made. On machines available to veterinary practice, up to three frames a second are possible. The images produced will be 'normal radiographs' with bone appearing white and lungs will be black. When setting up a fluoroscopy unit, the image intensifier should be as close to the patient as possible, preferable above the patient.

Uses of fluoroscopy

Fluoroscopy can be used anywhere that a real time (moving) image is needed. This includes barium swallow examinations (Figure 13.4), the removal of oesophageal foreign bodies and some interventional procedures such as angiography or portosystemic shunts. It can also be used during orthopaedic surgery to check the position of screws, but care must be taken with radiation safety when using it in this situation.

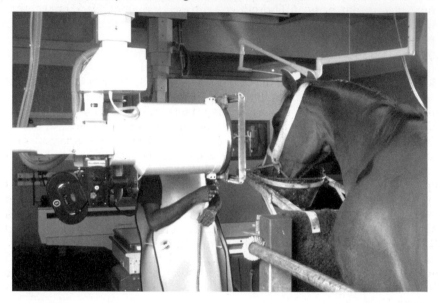

Figure 13.4. Fluoroscopy during a barium swallow of a horse.

Problems with fluoroscopy

The problems encountered with fluoroscopy are the same as those for general radiography including suitable sedation and positioning. There is, however, less of a problem with the dose received by staff and patients as the exposure is minimal. This does not, however, mean that safety precautions can be relaxed. Lead aprons must be worn at all times when fluoroscopy is being used.

Digital imaging

Digital imaging is becoming more common in radiography, although due to the cost it will be many years before it is found in general veterinary practice.

Digital imaging will produce a digital or numerical image. This has the advantage that images can be manipulated to give a diagnostic image, where repeat radiographs may be the only option with conventional imaging. The images can be stored on disk rather than on bulky film, reducing the storage necessary and can lead to film-less practice. A 'cassette' is still needed, but it contains a fluorohalide that is energized when exposed to X-rays rather than a film. Examinations are performed in the usual way and then retrieved from the fluorohalide through the use of a laser onto a computer where they can be manipulated.

Computerized tomography (CT)

This technique produces images of selected thin cross-sectional slices of the body. Conventional radiography produces images that are parallel to the long axis of the body; CT produces a transverse image (an image that appears to have sliced the patient from front to back).

How it works

A scout image is produced. This demonstrates the whole body and from this the areas for examination can be determined. The patient is examined from lots of angles by a thin X-ray beam using the principles of tomography. The X-ray tube and detector will move around the patient at one level and then the examination table will advance the patient through the scanner so a further slice at the next level can be acquired. At this stage no image is actually formed. The radiation that has passed through the patient is picked up by a detector and fed into a computer. This data is recorded as a series of numbers and is then reconstructed into a digital image by the computer and displayed on a monitor. This can then be manipulated to produce a diagnostic image. The images can then be stored on a disk or on normal X-ray-type film. The image is in the form of lots of small units called pixels. Each pixel has a numerical value known as a CT number. They are measured in Hounsfield units. Water has a Hounsfield unit of zero, air 1000 and muscle 50. All tissue types within the body will have different Hounsfield units (Figure 13.5).

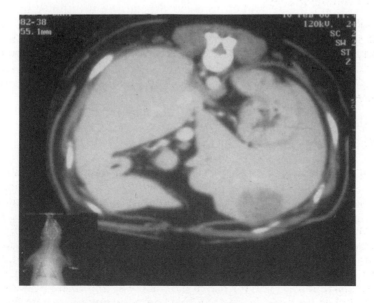

Figure 13.5. CT image of an abdomen.

Problems with CT

The only problems with this type of examination are:

1. The patient must remain still for the whole examination. Patient movement will result in a blurred image and inaccurate slices. Between slices the table will move the patient further through the scanner. This may cause movement if the patient is not adequately restrained using anaesthesia.
2. The usual safety considerations during the use of ionizing radiation need to be followed. This includes ensuring that only necessary people are in the room during exposures. Due to the nature of the examination this is usually for the entire acquisition period.

Uses

CT is useful in the diagnosis and staging of tumours and the diagnosis of central nervous system disorders. It can also be used to supplement any radiological examination where more detail is needed.

Magnetic resonance imaging (MRI)

MRI uses a magnetic field and the effect a certain radio frequency has on this field to produce a radio signal. This effect relies on the fact that tissues have nuclei, which produce different radio signals, dependent on their atomic number. When the patient is in the scanner a magnetic field is applied around their body. This makes all the atoms spin. A radio signal is then applied to the area and this makes the atoms relax back to their original position. The time it takes for this relaxation to occur depends on the atomic number of the nucleus. Different materials relax at different speeds and this determines the density on the image, which is produced by the computer system.

The big advantage of MRI is that it does not use ionizing radiation.

Problems with MRI

Due to the presence of the magnetic field and radio signal a number of precautions need to be followed.

- Patients with pacemakers or a new prosthesis must not enter the scanner room
- Credit cards and anything with a magnetic strip will be wiped if they are taken into the scanner room
- Metal objects should not be taken into the scanner room, as they will move very quickly towards the bore of the magnet. This includes scalpels, needles, oxygen cylinders or trolleys.
- A coil must be placed around the area under examination.This looks like a tube, but actually plays a vital role in applying the radio frequency.
- The scanner can be noisy.
- Examination times can be long and so anaesthesia is necessary to reduce patient movement.

Areas suitable for examination

MRI is more sensitive than CT for investigation of the nervous system. This includes the brain, and the associated blood and nerve supply. MRI will also demonstrate spinal cord lesions very well. MRI has very poor definition for bone and structures containing calcium, but is very good for associated muscle and joint composition. The technique is also very good for showing abnormalities in the thorax, including tumours and vascular anomalies. Contrast agents can be used to enhance the image if it is thought to have a blood supply (see Figure 13.6).

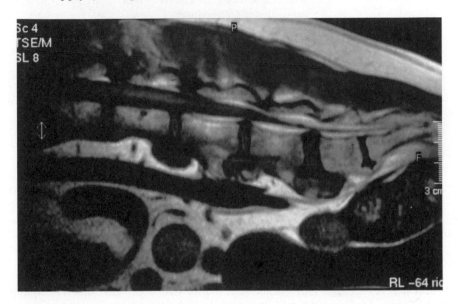

Figure 13.6. MRI image of the lumbar spine.

Ultrasound

Ultrasound is the use of very high frequency sound waves to produce a diagnostic image. These sound waves are above 20 000 Hz, which is well above the audible range of humans. Diagnostic ultrasound uses a range of 2.5–12 MHz (see Figure 13.7).

How ultrasound works

Ultrasound is formed in waves from a transducer. The transducer consists of a ceramic crystal between two pincers. A current is applied to the pincers, which will pass through the crystal and crush it. When the voltage is applied to the ceramic a pulse of high frequency sound waves is produced. The sound wave will pass through the body and then bounce back, causing compression of the ceramic and the creation of an electrical impulse. This is known as piezo-electricity. This can be repeated a number of times a second as the

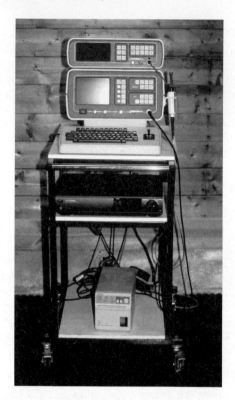

Figure 13.7. Ultrasound machine.

process is very quick. The speed of the ultrasound waves through soft tissues is 1540 m/s. The impulses are amplified and displayed on a monitor to give a continuous image. These can then be frozen and printed or recorded on a video as a moving image (real time) to be viewed at a later date.

Different tissues have different resistance levels to the passage of sound and this will alter the reflection of the sound waves back to the transducer. This will alter the appearance of the tissues on the image produced and allows differentiation between tissue types.

Image display modes

A Mode   The use of this is now limited. This uses a horizontal axis to show the depth into the patient of the tissue boundary and a vertical axis to show the strength of the echo.

B Mode   This is the most common mode in use today. The mode will use lots of scan lines from the source to produce a two-dimensional cross-section image. The image is changing all the time and allows the movement of structures to be seen.

M Mode   This is used in cardiology as it allows the movement of structures to be shown as a frozen image.

Effects on tissue

Ultrasound has not been shown to cause any long-term damage to tissue although research is still being carried out. It has, however, been shown to have some effect on tissues which do not cause long-term problems. Ultrasound will generate heat within the tissue and a micro-massaging effect. The combination of these two effects can be used in humans in a physiotherapy situation to benefit the patient. The ultrasound waves will also make all the electrons within the area of examination flow in the same direction and this effect is known as micro streaming.

Patient preparation

For the ultrasound examination to be effective, the animal must have the area prepared. This allows for the ultrasound waves to pass from the transducer into the patient and back again without interference from the air outside of the patient.

- The area for examination is clipped; areas with underlying bone or gas should be avoided, as this will block the movement of the sound waves
- Spirit is used to remove any residue dirt and grease on the skin surface
- Coupling gel is applied to the transducer and the skin to ensure contact between the skin and transducer without the interference of air

Areas suitable for examination

Ultrasound is becoming the examination of choice for the diagnosis of more and more diseases; however, it cannot replace all the tasks which radiography can perform. It is suitable for use in practices as it is mobile, easy to store and needs no specific precautions or areas for use. The main disadvantage is that operators need experience and if this experience is lacking diagnosis may be inaccurate.

The main areas of examination are abdominal soft tissue organs, the heart, thyroid, larynx, tendons, ligaments and soft tissue masses. It can also be used for pregnancy diagnosis, but is not accurate enough to determine numbers in small animals or sex.

Ultrasound can also be used as a means of guiding needles during biopsies, cytocentesis or fine needle aspirates.

Bone cannot be examined and may cause artefacts on the images of other regions if the ultrasound wave has to pass through or past bone to reach the area of interest. Large amounts of air can also obscure the area of interest and cause artefacts.

Nuclear scintigraphy

This type of examination uses a radioactive isotope attached to a compound that will be taken up by a certain substance in the body (e.g. bone, thyroid tissue) following injection into the circulatory system. After a set period of time the patient is placed in front of a detector and the amount of radiation emitted from certain points is recorded and evaluated against the expected normal values. In an area where there is an abnormality the isotope will either be present in a higher amount (hot spot) or not present at all (cold spot). The uptake can either be recorded on a hand-held probe giving counts at certain points or on a gamma camera, which will show the images on a monitor (see Figure 13.8).

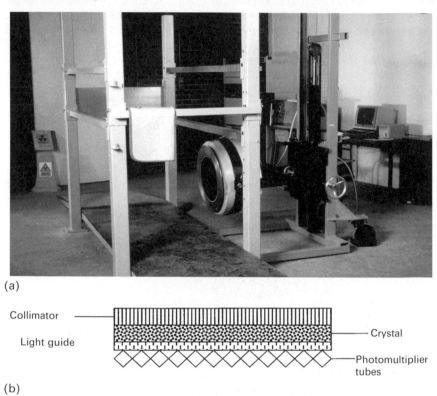

(a)

Collimator ——————

Light guide ——————— Crystal

———— Photomultiplier tubes

(b)

Figure 13.8. a, Gamma camera ready for an equine examination; b, structure of the collimator head.

The gamma camera

The gamma camera is the most accurate method of detecting the gamma radiation emitted by the patient. The camera consists of a large sodium iodide crystal. This will convert the gamma radiation to light. Photomultiplier tubes that convert the light into electrical pulses then detect the light. The photomultiplier tubes amplify these electrical pulses. The electrical pulses are counted by an electronic monitor and plotted on a television monitor to give a diagnostic image.

The front of the gamma camera has a collimator that acts in a similar way to a grid. It will remove all low energy gamma radiation and any radiation that is not moving in a forward direction. This will improve the quality of the resultant image.

Radiopharmaceuticals used

Radioisotopes are used in scintigraphy to provide the gamma radiation for detection. The isotopes are usually attached to a marker, depending on the organ to be examined. The most commonly used isotope in the veterinary field is Technetium^{99m}. The technetium has a half-life of 6 hours and an energy level of 140 keV, making it ideal for veterinary use.

Technetium can be attached to various compounds to allow it to target certain organs or body systems.

Hydroxymethylene Diphosphonate (HDP) will target bone; thyroid tissue as well as the stomach, and the salivary glands will take up technetium pertechnetate (see Figure 13.9).

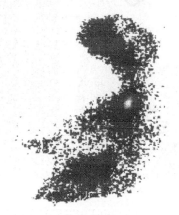

Figure 13.9. Thyroid scan of a cat with hyperthyroidism.

Problems with scintigraphy

There are two major problems when using scintigraphy:

- The patients need to be isolated for a minimum of 48 h after the isotope has been injected before it reaches a safe level. This means that the animal must be isolated for this period and that all their waste must be stored for the same period of time before it can be disposed of.
- The patient must be kept very still while the scan is performed. If they move the counts will produce a false image and this may lead to a misdiagnosis. Sedation must be good, but the animals must not wobble or sway if they are standing for the scan.

Regions suitable for investigation

Scintigraphy can be used to demonstrate bone in all animals. This will show stress fractures, tumours or other bony pathology. In cats it can be used to show the thyroid position and size. This is of diagnostic use because normal thyroid tissue will take up the radiopharmaceutical in similar amounts as the parotid salivary gland. If the thyroid is over active, this uptake will increase and the thyroid tissue will appear 'hotter' than the salivary gland. It can also be used to show kidneys, lungs and abdominal organs, but this use is limited in the veterinary field. Scintigraphy is also used in cases with suspected porto-systemic shunts to determine the fraction of blood bypassing the liver.

Revision points

- Tomography is the movement of the tube and film to blur out tissue above and below the object under investigation
- Tomography can be used to demonstrate kidney poles or the mandible
- Fluoroscopy provides an image that can be seen on a TV monitor as it happens (real time)
- The exposures required to produce a diagnostic image are very low
- Fluoroscopy can be used for barium swallow examinations, removal of foreign bodies or during interventional contrast examinations
- Digital imaging will provide a means of storing and manipulating images without the need for a radiographic film
- CT provides cross-sectional cuts of the body
- CT uses ionizing radiation and a detector
- CT can be used to demonstrate CNS disorders and tumours, and gives more detail than conventional radiographic examinations
- MRI uses a large magnet with a radio frequency being applied to produce an image
- MRI is ideal for the demonstration of soft tissue structures including the spinal cord, joints and the brain
- Ultrasound uses high frequency sound waves
- Ultrasound cannot be used where there are large amounts of gas or bone
- Nuclear scintigraphy uses a radioisotope
- The isotope is injected into the animal, attached to a marker and will be taken to the organ or system of interest
- Scintigraphy is mainly used for examination of the bone and the thyroid tissue in small animals

---

Revision questions

1. *In tomography what is the fulcrum?*
2. *Where can tomography be used?*
3. *Describe how an image intensifier works*
4. *Give three situations where fluoroscopy would be of use*
5. *If you were using digital imaging what would you not have to use?*
6. *Does CT produce transverse or longitudinal images?*
7. *Describe how atoms move during an MRI scan*
8. *What must you not take into an MRI scanner room?*
9. *Describe the patient preparation necessary for an ultrasound scan*
10. *What is the piezo-electric effect?*
11. *Name two substances that ultrasound waves will not image accurately*
12. *List three parts of the body that can be imaged using ultrasound*
13. *What are the parts that make up a gamma camera?*
14. *How does the radioisotope reach the structure of interest?*
15. *List two structures that can be imaged using nuclear scintigraphy*

14 Radiation protection

Introduction

Radiation safety should be remembered at all times when carrying out radiographic examinations. Adherence to the guidelines will ensure maximum safety for all personnel involved in diagnostic radiography. The guidelines are not designed to cause difficulties for the practitioner attempting to adhere to them, but to ensure their safety and protection. The biggest factor in radiation safety is distance. The greater the distance from the primary beam to an individual, the safer the situation.

The effects of ionizing radiation on the body

Ionizing radiation can originate from the X-ray tube or in the form of gamma rays. This radiation will damage cells and is not selective of cell type. The effects are more obvious in the immature or rapidly dividing cells. The amount of cell damage is determined by the amount of dose, the type of cell and its maturity. If the cell is still being formed when the dose is received then the DNA may mutate. Later in the cell cycle, repair may occur.

Biological effects	Heat, excitation and ionization
Cellular effects	Somatic, carcinogenic and mutation

Types of effect

Stochastic

This is a genetic effect. There is no safe dose and as the dose increases the chance of being affected increases.

Non-stochastic

This type of effect has a threshold level. Below the threshold, the chance of being affected is very low. Once the threshold is reached, the chance of being affected is very high.

Somatic

The person irradiated experiences these effects. This will occur during the lifetime of the person. These effects include skin reddening, blood disorders, cataracts or intestinal upset. These changes can happen very soon after exposure.

Genetic

With this type of effect, the effects of the radiation on the genetic make-up of the person may become apparent in future generations. The person receiving the dose will not be affected in their lifetime, however future generations may be.

Somatic stochastic

This is a cancer induced by the radiation and will be experienced during a lifetime. The effects may take time before they become evident.

Somatic non-stochastic

This effect of radiation can be used to our advantage in radiotherapy.

The basics to remember

Radiation protection has three basic principles that should be adhered to at all times. If these principles are always remembered then radiation safety will be maintained. The overall principle is known as the ALARA principle that should be adhered to at all times. This stands for As Low As Reasonable Achievable and can be maintained if the basics principles are remembered.

---

1. No dose limit should be exceeded.
2. Exposure to personnel should be kept to a minimum.
3. Unnecessary procedures should not be performed.

Ionizing radiation (medical exposure) regulations

The use of radiation and the law governing it was revised in 1999/2000 and is given in full in the document entitled *The Ionizing Radiation (Medical Exposure) Regulations 2000*. This gives all the information needed when using a source of radiation. The law also gives a number of regulations regarding maximum dose and control within the X-ray room.

All exposures used should be recorded along with patient details and stored with the machine. If there is no option but to manually restrain a patient then the holder must be documented with the exposures used.

There is also a publication especially for veterinary use of radiation entitled *Guidance Notes for the Protection of Persons against Ionizing Radiations arising from Veterinary Use*. This has specific guidelines for the veterinary practice.

Radiation safety in the veterinary practice

If the regulations laid out by the regulations are followed then the safety of patients and personnel is maximized.

To maintain the safety levels necessary, practices must carry out the following.

1. The health and safety executive (HSE) must be notified if the practice intends to start using X-rays. This ensures that the practice will be visited and inspected to ensure that safety levels are suitable.
2. The practice will need to appoint a Radiation Protection Supervisor (RPS). This is someone from within the practice who ensures that all the work is carried out safely.
3. A Radiation Protection Advisor (RPA) from outside the practice will be appointed. This person will help set up the working practices within the practice and set up the local rules.

Local rules

The local rules vary from one practice to another, but should ensure that:

- No animal is manually restrained
- No unnecessary personnel stay in the room during exposure
- Suitable protection is used
- Predetermined guidelines for pregnant members of staff
- Minimum age of 16 for trainee staff
- Areas within the practice are classified
- Guidelines for the implementation of warning signs during exposure

System of work

Details of this are prepared by the RPA and the RPS. This includes the Local Rules. These should be displayed where everyone can read them at any time. This is the legal responsibility of the RPS.

They should state:

- The name of the RPS
- A description of the restricted areas
- Details of access restriction
- Details of working practices
- Details of any plans should an incident occur

RPA	Radiation Protection Advisor
RPS	Radiation Protection Supervisor
Local Rules	Guidelines specific to the practice
Systems of work	Includes local rules and will give details of the area classification and the names of the RPA, RPS and any other important information relating to radiation safety

Classifying the areas around an X-ray machine

These areas are defined by the RPA and maintained by the RPS when X-rays are being taken.

Controlled area

A controlled area is the room in which the X-ray machine is positioned. The area is so designated when the amount of dose within the area exceeds 7.5 mSv/h. People who enter this area should be classified, with records kept of all the readings recorded from their monitoring devices.

The controlled area should have brick walls (stud walls do not provide adequate safety) and the room should be large enough to allow two people to stand at least 2 m from the tube. A warning sign should be placed at the entrance to the room and the number of people within the classified area kept to a minimum. This should be the radiation trefoil in black on a yellow background. An indication of when an exposure is being made is also compulsory either as a beep on the machine or a light outside the room (see Figure 14.1).

Supervised area

A supervised area surrounds the controlled area. This is any area that exceeds one-tenth of the recommended dose limit and therefore control of personnel entering this area needs to be monitored.

Dose limits

Dose levels are the amount of radiation received by an individual over a set period of time. These dose levels are controlled by legislation. They are

Figure 14.1. Example of a warning sign to be used outside of a controlled area.

designed to ensure that the dose received by personnel is kept to a minimum. If you ever need an X-ray yourself, you become a member of the general public at this point and not classified/trainee. You should not wear your monitoring device. The levels for classified personnel are designed to include not only people using diagnostic X-rays, but those using radiation in power stations and other industrial settings. These levels are decreasing each time the legislation is reviewed.

General public	5 mSv
Trainees (16–18 year olds)	15 mSv
Classified (over 18, with suitable training)	50 mSv

All doses must be recorded and transferred when staff move practices. The doses should be recorded using either a film badge or thermoluminescent dosimeter. Records of the exposures used for each case must also be recorded and kept. This record should be kept with the machine used or with the radiograph produced. The kV, mAs and distance used along with the film type and examination should always be recorded. It is also important to record any personnel who remained in the room during the exposure.

Monitoring devices

Monitoring devices are not compulsory, but advisable. The use of these ensures that personnel receive the minimum dose and anything that is received above this is known about. It will also ensure that the maximum does limits are not exceeded. The usual annual dose received by monitored personnel using diagnostic X-rays is approximately 2 mSv. To put this into context, background radiation in the UK is 1–2 mSv.

The readings from dosimeters are cumulative and will be maintained throughout the individual's career. Monitoring badges should not be shared by individuals and should be worn under protective clothing. This will give an accurate indication of the dose received by the body (rather than the dose received by the apron).

There are a number of different monitoring devices.

Film badge

A small film is placed in a plastic container. A number of different ports have varying thicknesses and types of metal. When the film is developed the degree of blackening on the film and the regions that are blackened will determine the dose received. The films are sent away for analysis and can only be used once making them expensive (see Figure 14.2).

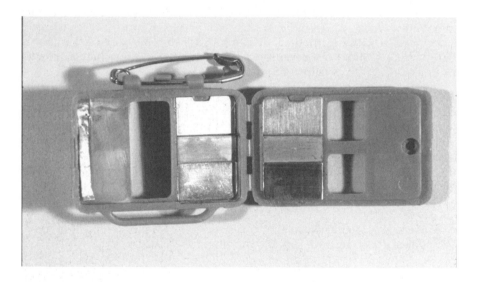

Figure 14.2. Open film badge.

Thermoluminescent dosimeter (TLD)

The dosimeter is of similar size to the film badge. It contains crystals of lithium fluoride, which has a similar density to soft tissues. After the dosimeter has been worn and possibly irradiated, it is heated and the amount of light emitted is compared to a standard, known, radiation dose. The dose received can then be calculated. This type of monitor can be re-used.

Lead shielding

If there is no alternative and personnel must remain in the room whilst an exposure is being made, lead protection must be used. This is usually in the form of a lead apron or a lead-lined screen. These contain a certain amount of lead and give protection against scattered radiation. This is measured in lead equivalent and is usually 0.5 mm for a lead apron. Lead shielding is only effective against scattered radiation. The energy levels in the primary beam are high enough to allow penetration through the lead. Scatter has low energy levels so it is absorbed by the lead.

Monitoring devices should be worn under the apron so that the dose received by the individual is accurately monitored. Lead aprons need to be checked from time to time to check for cracks that may reduce the protection received from the apron. Visual inspection will reveal any holes forming and even fairly small holes can be detected in this way.

In equine radiography if a film holder is used or the film is held during examination of the stifle, then lead gloves must be used by the individual as well as a lead apron.

All protection needs to be stored carefully. Folding is not advised as this may cause cracks or splits in the lead rubber. The ideal way to store an apron is hung up with no restrictions or compression on any part of the apron. Sheets of lead, gloves or sleeves should be stored flat again to prevent cracks from appearing (see Figure 14.3).

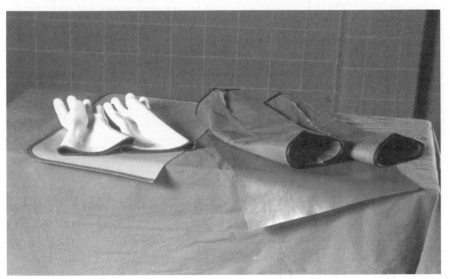

Figure 14.3. Lead shielding.

Quality assurance (QA)

QA forms an important part of the maintenance of a radiographic service and is an essential part of radiation protection. If QA is not carried out, there will be no baseline from which to determine any problems that may be present with the machine. QA covers both the X-ray machine and the processor. Both have an influence on the quality of radiographs being produced. Problems may occur with a machine and over time exposure factors are increased or altered to accommodate the changes. This is not good practice and through QA the problem can be detected before exposure factors are altered. For consistency, one individual should carry out QA.

X-Ray machine

QA can be carried out in practice on a routine basis as part of the annual service all equipment should receive. With the X-ray tube this should include checks on the filtration, the accuracy of the timer and the correspondence between the kV_p selected and what the tube is actually delivering. Specialist equipment is needed for these checks, which may be beyond the financial resources and technical abilities of the individual practice.

Light beam diaphragm checks

The accuracy of the light beam diaphragm can be checked within the practice very easily and can rectify disputes over collimation practice. The primary beam is collimated to a square about 5 cm smaller than the cassette. Paper clips are unwound and placed on the corners of the visible collimation. Using a low exposure, the film is exposed. This is then processed. On viewing the edge of the collimation should be at the same place as the paper clips. Any variation will demonstrate the inaccuracy of the collimators.

Processor

The QA necessary on a processor is varied, but should be carried out routinely, at least monthly. The rollers and tanks should be thoroughly washed with fresh running water. The temperature of the wash water and the developer should be checked, as these will influence the activity of the processing chemistry and the quality of the resultant image. Replenishment should be ongoing, as tired chemistry will reduce the effectiveness of the developing and fixing agents. Sensitometry and densitometry should be carried out to ensure the maintenance of constant processing conditions.

Revision points

- Ionizing radiation will damage cells
- Ionizing radiation is not selective of cell type
- Immature or rapidly dividing cells are at more risk of damage
- Dose limits should not be exceeded
- Exposure to personnel should be kept to a minimum
- Unnecessary procedures should not be performed
- The ionizing radiation (medical exposure) regulations [IR(ME)R] should be adhere to at all times
- The HSE should know that your practice has an X-ray machine
- Someone within the practice should be appointed as the Radiation Protection Supervisor (RPS)
- Someone with knowledge of radiation safety should be appointed as the Radiation Protection Advisor (RPA)
- Local Rules should be available for the practice
- A system of work should be devised for the individual practice
- A controlled area is the room in which the X-ray machine is being used
- The supervised area surrounds the controlled area
- Dose limits ensure that the dose received by personnel is kept to a minimum
- Monitoring badges record the amount of dose received by an individual
- There are two types – a film badge or a thermoluminescent dosimeter
- Lead shielding should be worn or used if it is essential that an individual remain in the controlled area during an exposure
- Quality assurance involves both the X-ray machine and the processor
- QA monitors changes to the equipment that may reduce radiation safety

Revision questions

1. *Give two forms of ionizing radiation*
2. *How will ionizing radiation affect cells?*
3. *What will be affected by the genetic effects of radiation?*
4. *What are the three basic principles associated with decreasing radiation exposure?*
5. *Which guidelines should be followed?*
6. *Who must be informed before a practice starts to use an X-ray machine for the first time?*
7. *What is the RPA?*
8. *Give three points that the local rules should include*
9. *Who devises the systems of work?*
11. *What type of walls should a controlled area have?*
11. *Where is the supervised area?*
12. *What is the minimum age of a classified worker?*
13. *How does a film badge record the dose received?*
14. *How does a TLD work?*
15. *List three QA tests or procedures that can be carried out easily by a practice*

15 Contrast media

Objectives
- Negative contrast medium
- Positive contrast medium
- Contrast examination procedures
- Gastrointestinal tract investigation
- Genito-urinary tract
- Myelography
- Other contrast examinations

Introduction

Contrast medium can be used to enhance structures that are not normally seen on plain radiography in detail or to outline cavities that may not be visible on plain radiographs. Contrast medium is divided into two distinct categories – positive and negative. Negative is usually air. This will appear black on radiographs. Positive contrast mediums include barium- and iodine-based compounds. Both of these will appear white on radiographs. Examinations using contrast medium should follow protocols so that vital information or projections are not excluded.

Negative contrast medium

Negative contrast medium is usually in the form of air, but can be oxygen, carbon dioxide or nitrous oxide. Air is the negative contrast medium of choice as it is cheap and readily available. Air will appear black on radiographs.

Air can be used in conjunction with positive contrast media to give a double-contrast study. Positive contrast can be used to coat any hollow structure. Air is then used to distend the structure. Air should be introduced after the positive contrast medium otherwise bubbles and uneven coating may occur. The positive contrast will cling to the lining and the air will highlight defects. This can be used in cystography and barium enema studies.

Positive contrast medium

All positive contrast medium is selected because it has a high atomic number. This increases the absorption of X-rays and will appear white on radiographs. The two types available are barium sulphate based and a water-soluble iodine compound.

Barium sulphate

This contrast medium is used to outline the alimentary tract. It is a white chalky powder that is mixed with water to produce a liquid suspension or a paste. It may be supplied as a ready-made colloidal suspension although this is not ideal if the use of the medium is limited in practice as once opened it is difficult to store.

Barium is completely insoluble and is not acted upon by digestive enzymes or absorbed by the intestine. Care should be taken, however, if it leaks into the peritoneum or is inhaled, as it may result in granulomatous adhesions or aspiration pneumonia. The barium may cause faeces to appear white and cause constipation (see Table 15.1).

Table 15.1. Barium sulphate preparations

Presentation	Proprietary Name	Manufacturer
Powder	Micropaque HD	Nicholas
	Baritop Plus	Bioglan
	E-Z-Paque	Henleys
Suspension	Baritop 100	Bioglan
	Micropaque standard	Nicholas

Iodine compounds

Iodine compounds used for contrast examinations are all water-soluble and appear as clear liquids. The water-soluble iodine compounds are usually used for all examinations other than those of the alimentary tract. They are not usually used for the alimentary tract unless perforation is suspected, as they are bitter to the taste, making it difficult to introduce them to conscious animals and do not give good contrast when compared with barium sulphate. They are usually more viscous than water and are very sticky. As they are water-soluble they can be injected directly into the vascular system. The contrast medium is excreted by the kidneys soon after injection and can therefore be used for examinations of the kidneys, ureters and bladder (see Table 15.2).

Water-soluble iodine compounds come in varying concentrations. The concentration is expressed as the amount of iodine per millilitre of medium. As an example Conray 420 will contain 420 mg of iodine in every millilitre. Depending on the area under examination a suitable concentration should be selected. This decision should take into consideration the amount of dilution that will occur after introduction.

> ## Concentration of water-soluble iodine compounds
> ... mg of iodine per millilitre of medium

Water-soluble contrast medium falls into two categories – ionic and non-ionic. Ionic contrast medium can cause adverse reactions including vomiting, irritation and anaphylaxis. These reactions are due to the high osmolar pressure of the contrast medium and the toxicity of the contrast medium on normal body fluids. These contrast mediums should only be used for introduction into cavities such as the bladder or intravenously in healthy patients.

If the patient is unwell or is under going myelography, more expensive non-ionic contrast mediums should be used. These have a lower osmolality and cause fewer side effects. Care should be taken to ensure that they are recommended for use during myelography.

Table 15.2. Water-soluble iodine preparations

Presentation	Ionic/non-ionic	Proprietary Name	Concentration (mg I/ml)	Manufacturer	Uses
Sodium iothalamate	Ionic	Conray 420	420	Mallinkrodt	IVUs angiography
Sodium/meglumine iothalamate	Ionic	Conray 280	280	Mallinkrodt	IVUs
Sodium/meglumine diatrozoate	Ionic	Urografin 150	150	Schering	Sinography, fistulography, bladder studies
Iopamidol	Non-ionic	Niopam 300/370	300/370	E Merck	All contrast studies except myelography
Iohexol	Non-ionic	Omnipaque 240/300/350	240/300/350	Nycomed Amersham	All examinations

Contrast examination procedures

To ensure maximum benefit from the expensive and time-consuming examinations a number of principles need to be remembered.

- Proper preparation of the patient should be ensured
- Adequate sedation or anaesthesia should be administered
- Preliminary radiographs should always be taken before the introduction of contrast medium – this will ensure suitable exposure factors are used and will demonstrate any abnormalities that may not be visible after the contrast medium has been introduced
- Adequate contrast medium of a suitable concentration should be given
- Any spillage should be removed immediately to prevent artefacts
- Positioning and collimation should be accurate

Gastrointestinal tract

Examination	**Barium swallow**
Use of examination	Used to outline the oesophagus
Indications	Regurgitation
	Retching/dysphagia
	Suspicion of foreign bodies
Patient preparation	None required
Sedation	Mild sedation if essential
	Barium should not be administered if the animal is heavily sedated or anaesthetized
Dose	Liquid barium sulphate suspension
	Dogs – 5–20 ml liquid depending on size
	Cats – up to 5 ml of liquid depending on size
	OR a small quantity of paste or barium mixed with food
	Do not use food if you want to follow the barium through from the stomach
Administration of contrast medium	Use a syringe in the corner of the mouth or allow the food or barium paste to be eaten – avoid spillage
Radiographic technique	• Plain lateral radiograph of the thorax before giving the barium
	• Thorax immediately after administration

Examination	**Barium meal and/or follow through**
Use of examination	To outline the stomach and duodenum
Indications	Vomiting
Patient preparation	No food for 12 h
	No water for 2 h
Sedation	Moderate sedation to allow multiple radiographic views to be taken
Dose	Liquid barium sulphate suspension
	Dogs – 1–3 ml/kg body weight
	Cats and very small dogs – 2–5 ml/kg body weight
Administration of contrast medium	By mouth with a syringe (some animals may drink the barium)
	Using a stomach tube – this ensures that no inhalation takes place and that the barium is introduced quickly in one dose.
Radiographic technique	• Preliminary plain lateral and ventrodorsal films of the abdomen should be taken
	• If fluoroscopy is available this can be used to watch the movement of the stomach
	• Four views of the stomach should be taken immediately after administration:
	(i) right lateral recumbency,
	(ii) ventrodorsal,
	(iii) left lateral recumbency and
	(iv) dorsoventral.
	This will ensure that all areas of the stomach are demonstrated

- Take ventrodorsal and right lateral recumbency films centred for the abdomen every 30 min until the stomach has emptied completely
- To demonstrate the small intestine, radiographs should be taken every hour after the stomach is empty

Examination	**Barium enema**
Use of examination	Used to demonstrate large bowel if proctoscopy is not available
Indications	Melaena
	Chronic diarrhoea
	Tenesmus
Patient preparation	The animal should be fed a low residue diet for 3 days
	A non-irritant enema should be administered 2–3 h before the examination to ensure that the bowel is empty
Sedation	General anaesthesia or very heavy sedation
Dose	Dilute liquid barium mixed 50 : 50 with warm water
	Approximately 10 ml/kg body weight
Administration of contrast medium	A bag containing the contrast medium and water should be hung from a drip stand
	A Foley catheter should be inserted into the rectum, attached to a rubber tube with a method of controlling the flow of barium (clamp is ideal)
	Barium should be allowed to flow slowly into the rectum by gravity

Radiographic technique

- Ventrodorsal and right lateral recumbency plain films of the abdomen should be taken
- Radiographs of the bowel should be taken after introduction of the barium in:
  - (i) right lateral recumbency,
  - (ii) left lateral recumbency and
  - (iii) ventrodorsal
- kV should be increased to penetrate the edges of the barium
- If a double-contrast enema is required, the barium should be removed from the colon, again by gravity
- Air should be introduced into the colon to make the barium cling to the mucosa and highlight any defects in the surface
- Radiographs should repeated with the kV reduced to prevent over exposure

Genito-urinary tract

Examination	**Intravenous urography (IVU)**
Use of examination	Used to demonstrate the function and anatomy of the kidneys and ureters

Indications	Incontinence
	Persistent haematuria
	Pyelonephritis
	Trauma
Patient preparation	Food should be removed for 12 h and water for 2 h before examination
	A cleansing enema should be given before the study as faeces in the colon may overly the kidneys and ureters
	The bladder should be emptied
Sedation	General anaesthesia is essential to prevent movement during the examination
Dose	Conray 420 – 1 ml/kg body weight
	Conray 280 – 2 ml/kg body weight
Administration of contrast medium	Rapid intravenous injection as a bolus
	OR a rapid drip infusion if a low concentration of iodine is being used (Urografin 150)

Radiographic technique

- Plain right lateral recumbency and ventrodorsal films centred on the umbilicus should be taken before introduction of the contrast
- From the end of injection:
    - (i) immediate ventrodorsal film at the level of the umbilicus,
    - (ii) 5 min ventrodorsal film at the level of the umbilicus,
    - (iii) 10 min right lateral recumbency film at the level of the umbilicus and
    - (iv) 15 min right lateral recumbency film centred at the level of the bladder neck
- More radiographs may be necessary if abnormalities are detected or excretion is slow.

Examination	**Urethrogram – male**
Use of examination	To demonstrate the bladder, urethra and prostate
Indications	Incontinence – may be used in conjunction with an IVU
	Dysuria
	Persistent haematuria
	Trauma
	Position of bladder
Patient preparation	A cleansing enema is useful, but not essential
Sedation	General anaesthesia is recommended but not essential
Dose	Urografin 150 or more concentrated contrast, diluted with sterile water
	Approximately 2 ml/kg
Administration of contrast medium	A small Foley catheter is introduced into the penile urethra and the cuff inflated to prevent the escape of the contrast medium
	The Foley catheter should be flushed with contrast before insertion to prevent the introduction of air bubbles

	Hands and forearms should be protected with lead gloves or sheets
Radiographic technique	• A plain film should be taken in right lateral recumbency, centred for the bladder neck and collimated to include the whole urethra
	• The bladder should then be catheterized and emptied
	• The animal should be repositioned as before
	• The contrast should be injected and the film exposed during the injection

Examination	**Urethrogram – female**
Use of examination	To demonstrate the bladder, urethra and vagina – may be used in conjunction with an IVU
Indications	Incontinence
	Dysuria
	Persistent haematuria
	Trauma
	Position of bladder
Patient preparation	A cleansing enema is useful, but not essential
Sedation	General anaesthesia is essential
Dose	Urografin 150 or more concentrated contrast, diluted with sterile water
	Approximately 1 ml/kg to fill the vagina and urethra
Administration of contrast medium	A small Foley catheter is placed in the vestibule of the vagina and the cuff inflated to prevent the escape of the contrast medium (the catheter is held in place and placing Allis tissue forceps across the vulva prevents back flow of the contrast – this can stimulate the animal and adequate anaesthesia is essential)
	The Foley catheter should be flushed with contrast before insertion to prevent the introduction of air bubbles
	Hands and forearms should be protected with lead gloves or sheets
	The contrast medium should be introduced in small increments, with the first film taken after two-thirds of the medium is introduced
	If the urethra is not full, then more contrast medium can be introduced
Radiographic technique	• A plain film should be taken in right lateral recumbency, centred for the bladder neck and collimated to include the whole urethra
	• The bladder should then be catheterized and emptied
	• The animal should be repositioned as before
	• The contrast should be injected and the film exposed during the injection

Examination	**Cystography**
Use of examination	Used to demonstrate the bladder
Indications	Dysuria
	Persistent haematuria
	Trauma
	Position of bladder
Patient preparation	A cleansing enema is useful, but not essential
Sedation	General anaesthesia is recommended but not essential
Dose	Pneumocystogram – air – 10 ml/kg body weight OR until the bladder feels distended
	Positive contrast cystography – Urografin 150 – 10 ml/kg body weight
	Double-contrast cystography – as for positive cystography, then remove contrast medium and replace with air
Administration of contrast medium	The bladder should be catheterized and urine removed
	The contrast medium or combination of contrast medium and air should be introduced slowly and if resistance is felt no further introduction should take place
Radiographic technique	• A plain film should be taken in right lateral recumbency, centred for the bladder neck
	• The bladder should then be catheterized and emptied
	• The animal should be repositioned as before
	• The contrast should be injected and the film exposed immediately after injection
	• For a pneumocystogram, the kV should be reduced

Myelography

Myelography is the introduction of positive contrast medium into the subarachnoid space around the spinal cord. The absence or deviation of the column of contrast medium surrounding the spinal cord will demonstrate lesions. Throughout this examination, speed is essential, as the contrast will be absorbed rapidly into the blood stream.

Indications	Spinal pain
	Paraplegia
	Quadriplegia
	Ataxia
	Trauma
Patient preparation	The contrast medium can be introduced through a cisternal or lumbar puncture. Whichever route is chosen, the area should be clipped and surgically cleaned to ensure sterility
Sedation	General anaesthesia essential
	Valium is often given just before the contrast is injected
Dose	0.3 ml/kg body weight of a non-ionic contrast medium up to 10 ml

Hexabrix should NOT be used – despite being of a low osmolarity it contains Ioxaglate, a mono-acid dimer, which is ionic, and not a suitable contrast medium for use during myelography.

Administration of contrast medium

Cisternal puncture. The head and shoulders should be raised 10° to prevent the contrast from flowing back into the ventricles of the brain. The head is flexed 90° to the neck. The spinal needle is inserted between the skull and the atlas until CSF drips from the needle. This should be collected in sterile containers for analysis. The contrast is injected slowly and the needle is then removed and the neck is extended.

Lumbar puncture. The spinal column is flexed by placing the front legs through the hind legs. This should not be done if there is any suspicion of instability of the spine. The needle is inserted at the level of the L4–5 or L5–6 junction. The hind legs will twitch as the needle passes through the spinal cord. Little or no CSF may appear and so a test radiograph will demonstrate the position of the needle and the contrast medium, before all of the contrast is introduced incorrectly. After introduction the needle is removed and the spine is extended. The head should be raised to prevent the contrast from flowing into the ventricles of the brain.

Radiographic technique

- Preliminary lateral radiographs should be taken to *demonstrate the area under suspicion*
- A test radiograph may be necessary with a lumbar puncture – this should be in lateral recumbency centred over the needle
- Lateral projections should be taken of the spine starting at the injection site and moving with the contrast
- If the contrast does not flow, traction may be necessary – tying a bandage around the maxilla, making a loop at the free end and hanging this with some heavy sandbags over the end of the table can achieve this.
- Once the contrast is at the area of interest ventrodorsal projections should be taken
- In cases with suspected thoracolumbar lesions, following a lumbar puncture the ventrodorsal projection should be taken immediately
- If the cervical spine is involved, the endotracheal tube should be removed for the ventrodorsal projection

Aftercare

The animal should be carefully monitored after myelography and the head should be kept raised until the animal has recovered fully from the anaesthesia

Other contrast examinations

Arthrography

This examination will demonstrate the joint cavity and the articular surfaces. Between 1 and 1.5 ml of a non-ionic contrast medium is introduced into the joint, and then radiographs are taken to demonstrate the position of the contrast. This is used mainly in the shoulder.

Portal venography

This is used to demonstrate the vessels within the liver. It will show whether the liver is receiving adequate blood flow and whether there are any anatomic abnormalities. It is the examination of choice for the diagnosis of a porto-systemic shunt.

At laparotomy, a vein in the jejunum is selected and a cannula inserted and tied in position. Between 5 and 10 ml of water-soluble iodine based contrast medium is introduced as rapidly as possible and a radiograph centred over the last rib is taken on completion of the injection.

Sinography and fistulography

This will demonstrate the tract of any discharging sinus and the presence of any foreign body present. Fistulography will demonstrate the presence and path of a fistula. A catheter is placed into the opening of the sinus tract or suspected fistula and secured in place. Contrast is then introduced, ensuring that there is no spillage or back flow. On completion of the injection or when resistance is experienced a radiograph is taken.

Angiography and venography

Both of these examinations will demonstrate the vascular system. The best images are obtained when the catheter and contrast is placed directly into the vein or artery under investigation. A radiograph should be taken immediately after the termination of the injection. Some examinations may require films every 1–2 seconds to give adequate demonstration of the region.

Sialography

Used to demonstrate the salivary glands. Uses a very fine needle inserted into the salivary duct and the introduction of 0.5–1 ml of high-concentration, iodine-based contrast medium.

Dacryocystorhinogram

This examination will demonstrate the nasolacrimal duct in cats and dogs. Contrast is introduced through one of the puncta in the eye.

Arthrography	joints
Portal venography	hepatic portal veins
Sinogram	sinus tract
Fistulogram	fistula
Angiography	arterial blood supply
Venogram	venous blood supply
Sialogram	salivary glands
Dacryocystorhinography	nasolacrimal ducts

Revision points

- Negative contrast medium can be air, oxygen, carbon monoxide or nitrous oxide
- It will appear black on radiographs
- Barium sulphate should not be given to anaesthetized or heavily sedated animals as inhalation may occur
- In double contrast studies, positive contrast must always be administered before negative contrast
- Positive contrast medium always has a high atomic number
- Positive contrast medium will appear white on radiographs
- Barium sulphate is used for investigation of the alimentary tract
- It is a white chalky powder that is mixed with water to give a liquid suspension
- Barium is insoluble
- Barium is not acted upon by digestive enzymes
- Water soluble iodine compounds are used for all other types of contrast examinations
- They are in the form of clear liquids
- The concentration is described in milligrams of Iodine per millilitre of medium
- Water soluble contrast medium is either ionic or non-ionic
- Non-ionic contrast medium is safe to use in all areas, but is more expensive
- Ionic contrast medium has a high osmolarity and should not be used for myelography or examination of very weak patients
- A protocol for each examination should be followed to ensure diagnostic examinations
- All contrast must be removed from the X-ray table and equipment after use to prevent artefacts from being seen on radiographs

Revision questions

1. Give two reasons why air is the negative contrast agent of use
2. What is a double-contrast study?
3. Why should contrast medium be introduced before air?
4. Describe a barium sulphate suspension
5. Why should barium sulphate not be given to anaesthetized or heavily sedated animals?
6. How are iodine-based compounds introduced?
7. How much iodine does Urografin 150 contain?
8. Why should non-ionic contrast medium be used when available?
9. How much barium would you use in a barium swallow on a dog?
10. For a barium swallow, what radiographs would you take?
11. During a barium follow through, how often should radiographs be taken after the stomach has emptied?
12. Describe how barium should be administered for a barium enema
13. List the patient preparation for an intravenous urogram
14. What is the approximate dose of contrast medium needed for an intravenous urogram in a border collie?
15. How often should radiographs be taken during an intravenous urogram?
16. During an urethrogram what protection should be used?
17. What will a double contrast cystogram demonstrate?
18. What type of contrast medium must be used for myelography?
19. What is the dose rate of contrast medium for myelography?
20. What is a sinogram?

16 Radiography techniques

Introduction

Once a full understanding of how an X-ray machine works and how manipulation of exposure factors influence the final radiograph is gained, then positioning will take on more meaning and can be used to produce a diagnostic and visually pleasing image. Through the use of a personal routine, the process of taking a radiograph can be efficient without missing vital stages that may have a detrimental effect of the image quality. At all times radiation safety must take priority over all other considerations.

General principles

To ensure maximum benefit from accurate positioning the following principles should be followed.

- Only films that are clinically indicated should be taken – 'for completeness', 'because the owner thinks...' or 'because it would be nice' are not acceptable reasons for a radiograph
- Radiation safety guidelines must be adhered to at all times.
- Standard projections should always be taken in the first instance – if this is not done, interpretation is more difficult and accurate diagnoses may not be possible

- Standard projections are always a pair of projections at 90° to each other – this prevents pathology from being missed, either by other structures overlying or the pathology only being visible in one projection
- Careful positioning, centring and collimation should be maintained at all times
- If a horizontal beam is being used, consideration should be given to the path of the primary beam after it has passed through the animal
- If the positioning will compromise the animal's condition careful consideration should be given to the outcome of performing the investigation
- Careful indexing and cross referencing should be in place so that films can be easily found and repeats are not performed as films are 'lost'

Restraint

To prevent the production of low-quality or non-diagnostic images, some means of restraint is usually necessary. At no time should an animal be held. Regardless of how ill the animal is, some means of chemical sedation or aids for restraint with patience, are all that are needed to get a diagnostic radiograph. Attempting radiographs with no sedation at all may result in a non-diagnostic image and a breakdown in the radiation safety practices being employed. This should be avoided at all times. Even very dyspnoeic animals can be given some sedation to prevent manual restraint and further distress which may result in collapse.

Examination of the spine, skull, pharynx, some contrast examinations, hip examinations and most fracture investigations should not be carried out unless the animal is anaesthetized. Even with heavy sedation positioning will not be accurate as there will still be some muscle tone causing rotation and possible misinterpretation.

Positioning aids

As well as chemical restraint, positioning aids can be used to produce carefully positioned diagnostic images. These aids should be available for all examinations. Care must be taken to prevent artefacts from the aids being seen on the radiographs. Positioning aids can also be a source of cross-infection and contamination so care must be taken to keep them clean. The radio-opacity of all aids should be known before use to prevent repeat radiographs from artefacts.

- Radiolucent foam or plastic troughs for dorsoventral or ventrodorsal projections.
- A selection of radiolucent foam wedges and blocks. These should be in a variety of shapes and sizes. The range should include 45° wedges, square blocks and strips of foam. These should be washed after any use and contact with contrast medium.

- A selection of long floppy sandbags. These should not be placed in the primary beam, as they will be seen on the radiograph.
- Hobbles or bandages. These can be used to tie limbs out of the way or to hold the mouth open during examination of the bullae. These should not be used unless the animal is anaesthetized.
- Skull box. This is a box with graduated holes to accommodate bars for holding the patient in position when imaging the bullae or frontal sinuses.
- Positioning blocks and film holders are essential for equine examinations.
- A rope head collar is needed to prevent artefacts from being seen when imaging the equine head.

Markers and legends

All films should have anatomical markers that indicate the limb, the recumbency or the side of the patient. Markers should be placed so that they fall just outside the primary beam. This ensures that they are not over the region of interest but are seen in the scatter at the edges of the image. In equine work, the lateral aspect of the distal extremities should be marked so that lesions can be orientated. If films are part of a contrast examination, preliminary films and timed films should be marked. Markers come in a number of forms. The most common are metal clips or plastic tablets with the lead letters or markers embedded in the plastic. Whichever type is used, they will provide a permanent mark on the film.

All radiographs should have a permanent mark of the animals and owner's names, and the date of examination. This can be in the form of X-rite tape or through a marker that exposes the film with the details after exposure to the X-rays, but before processing. This is known as an actinic marker. It is simple to use and provides a readable and permanent means of identification.

Pre- and post-exposure labelling

All radiographs should be labelled prior to processing. This can be either during the exposure using X-rite tape or after exposure using an actinic light marker.

X-Rite tape is a special tape that when the details are written on it will allow them to be seen on the radiograph after processing. The tape strip must be in or close to the primary beam to be effective.

An actinic light marker will photograph the patient details onto the film after exposure but prior to processing. This uses a small light source to photograph the patient details onto the film. An area must be screened off on the film to allow this marker to be effective.

All films should have a minimum of the date and the patient details. A label added after processing is likely to fall off over time or be rubbed of the film.

Assessing the radiograph

When assessing a radiograph the following points must always be considered.

- Identification present and correct
- Markers and legends visible and correct
- Area under examination shown
- Correct projection taken
- Suitable exposure factors used for area under examination
- Adequate contrast, density and sharpness
- Collimation visible but not too tight
- Artefacts
- Any anatomical variants or gross pathology present that may alter exposure factors
- Good image quality
- Need for further projections or repeats

Terminology

All X-rays are described in terms of the path of the X-ray beam through the animal towards the film. It may also tell you how the animal was lying on the table. If an animal was lying with its right side on the table it is a right lateral recumbent film. This film will be marked as a 'right' lateral. Some projections are at an angle and this will also be added into the description of the projection. This is done most commonly in equine examinations (see Table 16.1).

Table 16.1. Terminology and abbreviations used in radiography

Full description	Abbreviation	Direction of X-ray beam or description or area
Left	L	
Right	R	
Dorsal	D	Front of lower limbs or top of main trunk
Ventral	V	Underside of animal
Cranial	Cr	Towards the head
Caudal	Cd	Towards the tail
Rostral	R	Towards the nose
Medial	M	Inside of leg
Lateral	L	Outside edge of legs
Proximal	Pr	The higher end of an extremity or bone
Distal	Di	The part of a bone or limb, furthest from the main body
Palmar	Pa or P	Back edge of the lower fore limb
Plantar	Pl	Back edge of the lower hind limb
Oblique	O	
Lesion orientated oblique	LOO	An oblique projection to skyline a lesion

British Veterinary Association/Kennel Club hip dysplasia and elbow scoring scheme

For both of these schemes set protocols should be followed. These are outlined below. Every animal undergoing these procedures must be over the age of 1 year and must have a kennel club certificate. Once taken the radiographs and relevant paperwork should be sent to the British Veterinary Association for scoring. Each breed has a specific score and the aim of the scheme is to minimize dysplasia by not breeding from animals with poor hips.

1. All animals must be over 1 year of age and have a Kennel Club certificate
2. The dog should be anaesthetized and placed in dorsal recumbency with the hind limbs extended so that the femora are parallel to the table top
3. The stifles should be rotated inwards and a tie placed just above them to hold them in place – sandbags and troughs may be needed to obtain good positioning
4. The Kennel Club registration number, the date and a left or right marker must be radiographed onto the film before processing – nothing should be added to the film after processing.
5. The films are then sent away for scoring, after which a written report will be sent to the veterinary surgeon and the owner

Positioning outlines – small animals

Chest

Right lateral recumbency (Figure 16.1)

- Forelegs extended and sandbagged
- Pad under sternum
- Sandbag to hold hind legs and neck
- Centre midway between the sternum and the spine, level with the caudal border of the scapula
- Collimate to include the front of the shoulder and the edge of the sternum
- Expose on inspiration

Dorsoventral chest (Figure 16.2)

- Patient placed in dorsal recumbency
- Chin supported on a pad
- Sandbag over the neck
- Forelegs pulled forward and adducted
- Centre at the midline at the caudal prominences of the scapulae

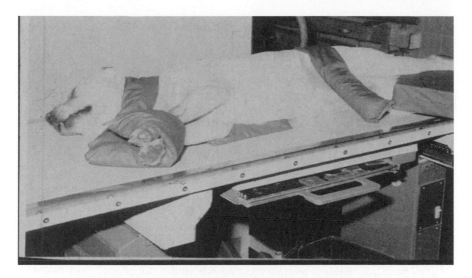

Figure 16.1. Positioning and restraint for a lateral chest.

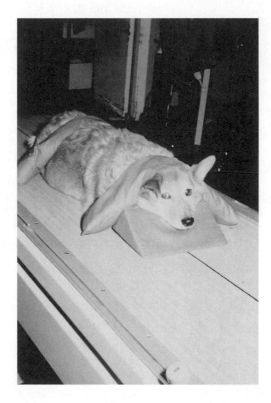

Figure 16.2 Positioning and restraint for a dorsoventral chest.

- Collimate to include the thoracic inlet and diaphragm
- Expose on inspiration

Abdomen

Right lateral recumbency

- Fore and hind legs sandbagged
- Pad under sternum
- Centre at the 11/12th intercostal space, just cranial to the last rib
- Collimate to include diaphragm and symphysis
- Expose just after expiration

Ventrodorsal abdomen (Figure 16.3)

- Patient placed in dorsal recumbency
- Sandbags over carpi
- Ensure that there is no rotation
- Centre on the midline at the level of the umbilicus
- Collimate to include diaphragm and symphysis
- Expose just after expiration

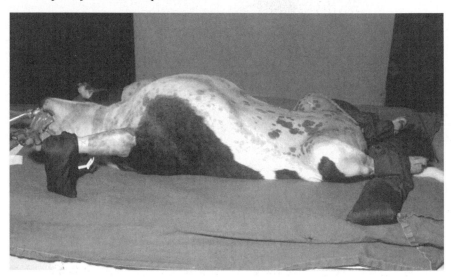

Figure 16.3. Positioning and restraint for a ventrodorsal chest or abdomen.

Head and neck

Ventrodorsal skull (Figure 16.4)

- The patient is placed in dorsal recumbency and the neck is extended
- A foam pad is placed under the neck to ensure that the hard palate is parallel to the cassette

- Centring is on the midline to include the area of interest (entire skull or tympanic bulla area)

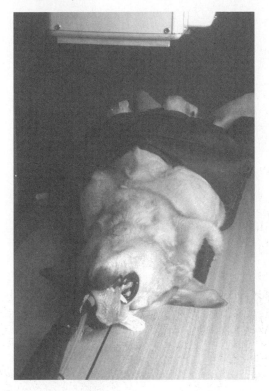

Figure 16.4. Positioning for a ventrodorsal skull.

Open mouth rostrocaudal view (tympanic bullae) (Figure 16.5)

- The patient is placed on its back with the hard palate perpendicular to the cassette
- The mouth is held wide open with tapes
- The beam is parallel to the hard palate centred on the base of the tongue
- The animal must have the endotracheal tube removed to demonstrate tympanic bulla adequately

Rostrocaudal view (frontal sinuses)

- The patient is placed on its back with the hard palate perpendicular to the cassette
- The beam is parallel to the hard palate centred on the middle of the nose
- Collimation should include the area of the frontal sinuses

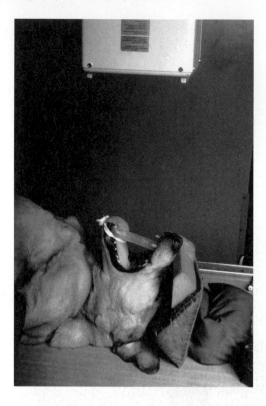

Figure 16.5. Positioning for an open mouth rostrocaudal view.

Dorsoventral intra-oral view (nasal chambers) (Figure 16.6)

- The patient is supported in sternal recumbency with the neck extended
- Place sandbag over the neck to prevent rotation
- Place a non-screen film into the mouth, corner first as far into the mouth as possible
- Centre the beam on a line midway between the external nares and a line joining the eyes
- Ensure that an anatomical marker is included

Nasopharynx (Figure 16.7)

- The patient is placed in lateral recumbency
- A pad supports the skull in a true lateral position and a pad is placed under the neck
- The legs are pulled caudally against the wall of the thorax
- Centring is at the mid-cervical area to include the pharynx and thoracic inlet
- The patient should be extubated prior to exposure

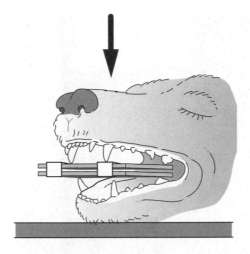

Figure 16.6. Positioning for a dorsoventral intra-oral view.

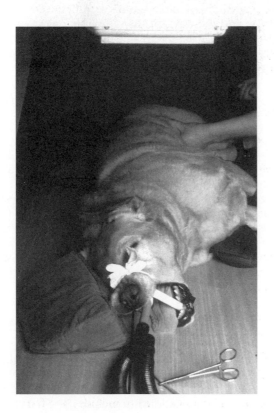

Figure 16.7. Positioning for a lateral nasopharynx.

Lateral oblique skull (temporomandibular joints, tympanic bullae)

- The patient is placed in lateral recumbency
- The fore legs are pulled caudally against the chest wall and held with a sandbag
- A pad is placed under the nose to raise it by approximately 30°. This will separate the temporomandibular joints or the bullae so that they can be seen more easily
- Centring is directly over the uppermost temporomandibular joint or tympanic bulla and collimation should include a small area around the area of interest
- The side nearest the film should be area under investigation
- Both sides need to be imaged for comparison

Oblique projection of the teeth

- The patient is placed in lateral recumbency
- A gag is placed in the mouth to separate the mandible and the maxilla
- The head is rotated slightly to remove the arcade nearest the tube away from the teeth under examination
- The teeth under examination should be seen between the upper arcade nearest the tube and the teeth of the mandible or maxilla
- Centring is on the last visible part of the tooth next to the gums
- Collimation should demonstrate the arcade from the temporomandibular joint to the midline of the head

Distal extremities

Mediolateral

- The patient is placed with the side to be imaged nearest the cassette
- The opposing limb is placed and supported on the flank (fore limbs pulled caudally, hind limbs pulled cranially)
- The limb should be parallel with the cassette – a pad may be necessary to prevent rotation
- Stifles and elbows should be flexed
- Centring is at the level of the joint or mid shaft
- Collimation is to include a joint above and below the long bone or a small area above and below the joint under investigation

Dorsopalmar/plantar and caudocranial
Horizontal beam (Figure 16.8)

- The patient is placed with the limb under investigation uppermost
- This limb is extended fully and supported with a pad so that it is parallel with the cassette
- Centring is at the level of the joint or mid shaft
- Collimation is to include a joint above and below the long bone or a small area above and below the joint under investigation

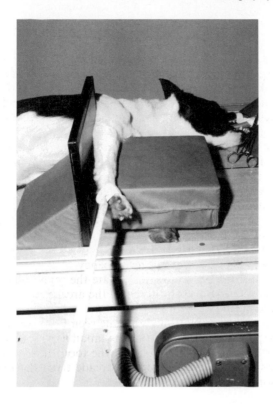

Figure 16.8. Positioning of an extremity using a horizontal beam.

Normal beam

- Patient is placed in sternal or dorsal recumbency so that the limb under investigation is parallel with the cassette
- The opposing limb may need to be lifted to rotate the limb under investigation so that it is straight
- Centring is at the level of the joint or mid shaft
- Collimation is to include a joint above and below the long bone or a small area above and below the joint under investigation

Shoulder

Lateral

- The animal is placed in lateral recumbency with the limb to be radiographed nearest to the cassette
- The head and neck are extended with sandbags
- The upper limb is retracted and secured with sandbags
- The limb under examination is drawn forward and ventrally
- The beam is centred at the level of and caudal to the lateral tuberosity

Caudocranial

- The patient is placed on its back and supported with sandbags – the thorax may need to be rotated slightly
- The affected limb is drawn cranially, fully extended and secured with a tie
- The beam should be centred level with acromion process

Pelvis

Ventrodorsal (Figure 16.9)

- The patient is placed in dorsal recumbency ensuring that the body is straight
- The hind limbs are extended so that the femora are parallel and rotated medially
- The hind limbs are tied above the stifles with sandbags over the stifles and hocks to maintain position
- The beam is centred at the level of the greater trochanter along the midline
- If the patient has a suspected fracture a frog leg view may provide the necessary information.
- The patient is placed on their backs and the legs are allowed to flop to the side to give the impression of a frog!

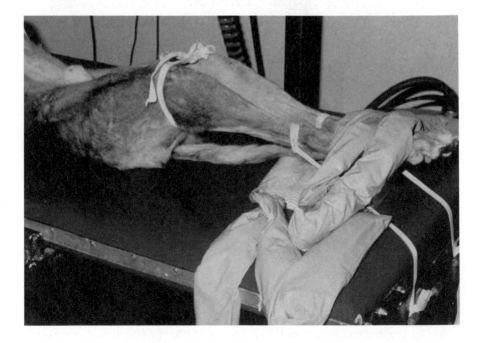

Figure 16.9. Positioning for a ventrodorsal pelvis.

Lateral pelvis
- The patient is placed in lateral recumbency
- Pads are placed between the hind legs to ensure that the pelvis is not rotated
- The beam is centred over the greater trochanter and collimated to include the entire pelvis

Spine

Lateral (Figure 16.10)

- The patient should be placed in lateral recumbency
- The spine should be supported with foam pads so that it is parallel with the tabletop
- Pads should be placed under the sternum and between the limbs to prevent rotation
- For the cervical spine the fore limbs should be pulled caudally
- The beam should be centred over the area of interest – if the entire spine is being examined, each image should overlap with the ones either side

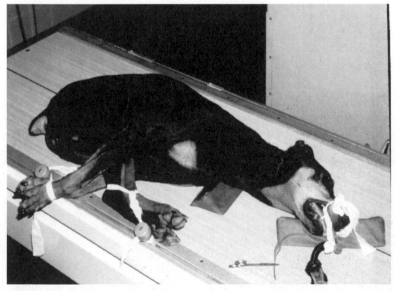

Figure 16.10. Positioning using sandbags and pads ready to centre for a spinal radiograph.

Lumbar sacral junction

Lateral

- This position has very specific positioning landmarks
- The greater trochanter of the femur should be identified and the cranial part of the ilial wing

- An imaginary line is drawn between the two landmarks. Centering is on the mid-point of the lines. Collimation should include both landmarks.

Ventrodorsal

- The animal is placed on its back supported in a trough or with sandbags
- The patient should be as straight as possible
- The hind legs should be extended to prevent rotation
- The beam should be centred over the region of interest

Positioning outlines – large animals (horses and cattle)

Foot

Dorsopalmar of the pedal bone (DPr60⁰–PaDiO)

- The foot should be clean and trimmed with the shoes removed.
- The frog should be packed to remove gas shadows – this packing material can be soap or playdough or other similar material
- The film is placed in a film holder and the foot placed on top of this
- The primary beam is centred below the coronary band on the midline of the foot with a downward angle of 60°
- Collimation should include the edges of the hoof wall and the toe and heel of the foot

Dorsopalmar of the navicular bone (DPr60⁰–PaDiO)

- The foot should be clean and trimmed with the shoes removed
- The frog should be packed to remove gas shadows
- The film is placed in a film holder and the foot placed on top of this
- The primary beam is centred just above the coronary band on the midline of the foot with a downward angle of 60°
- Collimation should be large enough to include all of the navicular bone

Lateromedial of the pedal bone and navicular bone

- The foot is prepared as for the dorsopalmar projection
- The foot is placed on a block to ensure that it is high enough off the ground
- The horse should be weight bearing on the limb
- The beam is projected parallel with the floor and centred at the level of the coronary band to include the heel and toe
- Collimation should include the weight-bearing surface of the foot
- If laminitis is suspected, a lead strip, the top level with the coronary band, should be placed down the midline of the hoof wall

Palmaroproximal–dorsodistal oblique of the navicular bone (Pa45Pr–DDiO)

- The foot is cleaned and trimmed and the frog is packed to remove any gas shadows
- The foot is placed on a film holder containing the film
- The foot is placed as far back as possible without the horse taking a step

forward – this removes the fetlock from the area of interest
- The X-ray beam is directed proximal to distal 30°–40° depending on how far back the foot is placed
- The beam is centred parallel with the long axis of the horse's leg and centred in the middle of the groove between the bulbs of the heel
- Collimation should be limited to the area of the navicular bone

Fetlock

Dorsopalmar

- The horse should stand, weight bearing on all feet
- The primary beam is angled down about 15° to ensure that is passes through the joint space
- The film is placed in a film box (Figure 16.11), behind the leg
- The beam is centred on the articulation of the fetlock passing along the midline of the leg
- Collimation should include the joint and a small area above and below the joint

Lateromedial

- The horse should stand, weight bearing on all feet
- The cassette is placed on the medial aspect of the leg, parallel with the leg
- The X-ray beam is centred on the articulation of the joint, parallel with the film
- Collimation should include a small area above and below the joint

Dorsolateral–palmaromedial oblique (D45L–PaMO) and dorsomedial–palmarolateral oblique (D45M–PaLO)

- The horse should stand, weight bearing on all four legs
- The primary beam is directed perpendicular to the leg
- For the DLPMO the cassette is placed midway between the medial and palmar surfaces of the leg
- For the DMPLO, the cassette is placed midway between the lateral and palmar surfaces of the leg – if the horse is not co-operating then a PLDMO is a safer projection to attempt as the X-ray tube and machine is not under the horse
- The X-ray beam is centred on the articulation of the joint

Cannon and splint bones

Dorsopalmar

- The horse should stand, weight bearing on all feet
- The film is placed in a film box or holder, behind the leg

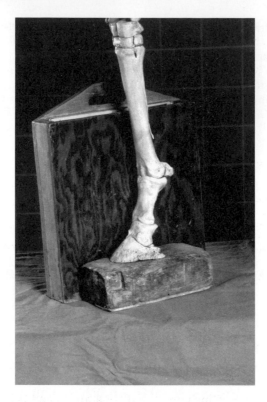

Figure 16.11. The use of a film box in the imaging of the distal limb of a horse.

- The beam is centred on the middle of the cannon bone along the midline of the leg
- Collimation should include the joints above and below the cannon bone

Lateromedial

- The horse should stand, weight bearing on all feet
- The cassette is placed on the medial aspect of the leg, parallel with the leg
- The X-ray beam is centred on the centre of the cannon bone, parallel with the film
- Collimation should include the joints above and below the cannon bone

Dorsolateral–palmaromedial oblique (D45L–PaMO) and dorsomedial–palmarolateral oblique (D45M–PaLO)

- The horse should stand, weight bearing on all four legs
- The primary beam is directed perpendicular to the leg
- For the DLPMO, the cassette is placed midway between the medial and palmar surfaces of the leg.
- For the DMPLO, the cassette is placed midway between the lateral and

palmar surfaces of the leg – if the horse is not co-operating, then a PLDMO is a safer projection to attempt as the X-ray tube and machine is not under the horse
- The X-ray beam is centred on the centre of the cannon bone, parallel with the film
- Collimation should include the joints above and below the cannon bone
- If the splint bones are under examination the oblique views should be taken with a reduced exposure

Hock and carpus (Figure 16.12)

Dorsopalmar

- The horse should stand, weight bearing on all feet
- The film is placed in a film box or holder, behind the leg
- The beam is centred on the middle of the joint passing along the midline of the leg
- Collimation should include the joint and a small area above and below

Lateromedial

- The horse should stand, weight bearing on all feet
- The cassette is placed on the medial aspect of the leg, parallel with the leg
- The X-ray beam is centred on the middle of the joint, parallel with the film
- Collimation should include a small area above and below the joint
- When imaging the hock, a slight angulation (10°) will improve image quality by allowing the primary beam to pass through the joint space

Dorsolateral–palmaromedial oblique (D45L–PaMO) and dorsomedial–palmarolateral oblique (D45M–PaLO)

- The horse should stand, weight bearing on all four legs
- The primary beam is directed perpendicular to the leg
- For the DLPMO, the cassette is placed midway between the medial and palmar surfaces of the leg.
- For the DMPLO, the cassette is placed midway between the lateral and palmar surfaces of the leg – if the horse is not co-operating then a PLDMO is a safer projection to attempt as the X-ray tube and machine is not under the horse
- The X-ray beam is centred on the middle of the joint

Elbow

Craniocaudal

- The horse should stand, weight bearing on all legs
- The limb under examination should be moved forward slightly to free it from the chest wall

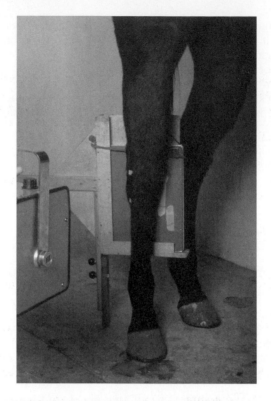

Figure 16.12. Positioning for an oblique projection of the hock.

- The head should be turned away from the leg to free it from the chest wall
- The cassette is angled and pushed up behind the elbow into the chest wall
- In larger animals a slight downward angulation may be necessary or angulation of the beam from medial to lateral
- The primary beam is centred on the distal margin of the humerus
- Collimation should include a small amount of the radius and the humerus

Lateral

- The film should be placed in a bucky or in a bag on a drip stand
- The affected leg is placed next to the film with the horse standing
- The leg under examination is then lifted forward and raised to reduce superimposition of the unaffected leg
- The primary beam is centred on the joint parallel with the film
- The person lifting the limb should wear lead protection

Shoulder

Lateral

- The film should be placed in a bucky or in a bag on a drip stand
- A grid should be used
- The affected leg is placed next to the film with the horse standing
- The leg under examination is then lifted forward and raised to reduce superimposition of the unaffected leg
- Raising the leg will also place the trachea over the joint, which will improve the image quality
- The primary beam is centred on the joint parallel with the film
- The person lifting the limb should wear lead protection

Stifle

Lateromedial

- The horse should have some contact around the stifle area before the examination begins
- The horse should be weight bearing on all legs
- A cassette is placed on the medial side of the horses leg and rotated up as high as possible
- This cassette is held and so adequate lead protection must be used
- The long edge of the cassette should be visible on the cranial edge of the leg
- The primary beam should be perpendicular to the cassette and the leg
- The primary beam is centred at the base of the patella
- The caudal aspect of the leg is not needed within the collimation as it only contains soft tissue

Caudocranial

- The horse should have some contact around the stifle area before the examination begins
- The horse should be weight bearing on all legs
- A cassette is placed on the cranial side of the horse's leg and lifted as high as possible
- This cassette is held and so adequate lead protection must be used
- The long edge of the cassette should be visible on the lateral edge of the leg
- The primary beam should be angled downwards about $10°$ so that it passes through the joint space
- The primary beam is centred at the base of the patella

Head

In the horse, imaging of the skull in the conscious patient is limited to a lateral projection. Further views can be taken under anaesthesia, but details will not be given here.

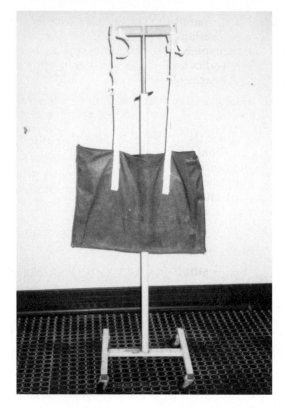

Figure 16.13. Film supported in a bag on a drip stand.

Lateromedial skull and sinuses

- The film is placed in a bag hung on a drip stand (Figure 16.13)
- A grid is not needed
- The horse stands with the affected side against the film holder
- A rope head collar should be used to prevent artefacts from buckles and clips
- The head is supported with a gloved hand
- The primary beam is centred at the base of the facial crest perpendicular to the head and film
- Collimation should include all of the maxilla, the frontal sinuses and the first cheek tooth

Spine

The spine of a horse can be easily imaged using a lateral projection with the horse standing. This is possible in general practice for the entire spine apart from the lumbar spine, beyond the diaphragm. The lumbar spine can be imaged but there is increased scatter reducing the image quality and a high mAs is essential.

The horse should stand, parallel to the film. Positioning should be over the spine and include some overlap from film to film so that all articulations can be assessed. The thoracic spine should be radiographed in two separate parts – one for the vertebral bodies and one for the spinous processes (withers). A grid is essential for all images of the spine

Chest

- Imaging of the equine thorax needs to be carried out in four parts – the exposure factors should be increased for cranial images due to the increase in tissue density
- Collimation should be no bigger than the film used
- All projections are laterals
- If an image is to be diagnostic either a grid or the air-gap technique should be used

Positioning outlines – small mammals, birds and reptiles

Small mammals (Figure 16.14)

- All small mammals can be radiographed without a grid
- Short exposure times can be used
- A film giving high definition is ideal
- The animal can be imaged in either lateral or dorsal recumbency; whichever keeps the animal the stillest

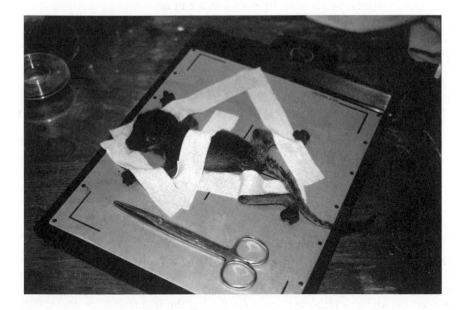

Figure 16.14. Imaging a small mammal.

Rabbits and guinea pigs

- For rabbits and guinea pigs a trough and sandbags can be used in a similar way to imaging a small cat or dog.
- With adequate sedation they will remain still using only these restraints.

Mice, gerbils and hamsters

- Smaller mammals may need to be placed into a Perspex tube or a roll of exposed X-ray film to keep them contained and in position.
- Tape may be used to position the animal although care must be taken to prevent them struggling and causing further injuries.

Birds (Figure 16.15)

Depending on the size of the bird, individual regions or the entire animal may be imaged.

Whole bird – ventrodorsal

- If the whole bird is to be imaged, it should be placed in dorsal recumbency on the cassette
- The wings should be extended to remove them from the body
- The legs should be drawn caudally
- The bird must be symmetrical to allow interpretation
- The wings, neck and legs must be secured with tape

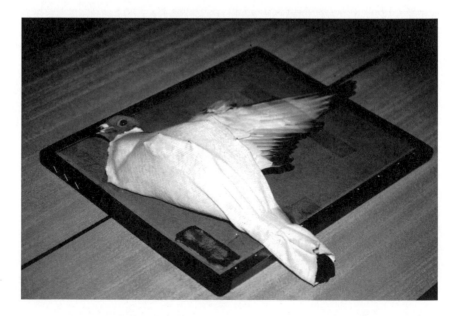

Figure 16.15. Positioning for a lateral projection of a bird.

Whole bird – lateral

- The bird should be placed in lateral recumbency
- The wings should be extended above the body and taped into position
- The legs should be secured to improve imaging (if the legs are the area of interest) and to restrain the bird

Reptiles

- It is possible to radiograph reptiles without sedation if they are allowed to cool to room temperature and their heads are covered
- No reptile will tolerate lateral recumbency and so a horizontal beam will be necessary if a lateral projection is required
- Restraint can be achieved using a Perspex box or tube or through the use of tape. Restraint may not be necessary however for many of these animals
- If the animal is too long to be fitted onto one film, multiple films can be used with overlap to ensure total coverage

Reading list

Ball J. and Price T. (1989) *Chesneys' Radiographic Imaging*, 5th Edition, Blackwell Scientific Publications.

Bryan G. (1987) *Diagnostic Radiography*, 4th Edition, Churchill Livingstone.

Burns F., Whelehan P. and Latham C. (1997) Understanding radiography: 3, *Veterinary Practice Nurse* **9**(2), 15–21.

Bushong S. (1997) *Radiological Science for Technologists* 6th Edition, Mosby.

Clarke K. and White R. (1998) Nursing the exotic patient, *Veterinary Nursing* **13**(4), 124–132.

Creighton D. (2000) Radiography case study. *Veterinary Nursing* **15**(3), 102–106.

Davies J. (1990) Improve your image. Part 1: X-Ray machines, *Equine Veterinary Education* **2**(1), 48–50.

Davies J. (1990) Improve your image. Part 3: Practical radiation safety, *Equine Veterinary Education* **2**(3) 151–154.

Dennis R. (1998) A scheme to control hip dysplasia. *Veterinary Nursing* **13**(2), 55–60.

Dennis R. (1997) Veterinary diagnostic imaging: into a new era, *The Veterinary Nursing Journal* **12**(2), 43–52.

Dennis R. (1987) Radiographic examination of the canine spine, *Veterinary Record* **121**(2), 31–35.

Dyson S. (1990) Current nomenclature relating to radiographic projections, *Equine Veterinary Education* **2**(3), 161–162.

Farrow C. (1981) Radiography of the equine thorax: anatomy and technic, *Veterinary Radiology* **22**(2), 62–68.

Ford G. (1999) Processing radiographs, *Veterinary Nursing* **14**(5) 187–188.

Guthrie S. (1996) Confused over calculations? Part 2: Radiography, *The Veterinary Nursing Journal* **11**(6), 190–191.

Harcourt-Brown F. (1998) Pet rabbits, *Veterinary Practice Nurse* Autumn 1998, pp. 4–6.

Head D. (1996) Risk assessment, *The Veterinary Nursing Journal* **11**(5), 142.

Jeffcott L. and Kold S. (1982) Radiographic xxamination of the equine stifle, *Equine Veterinary Journal* 14(1), 25–30.

Kirberger R. and Roos C. (1995) Radiographic artefacts, *Journal of the South African Veterinary Association* **66**(2), 85–94.

Latham C. (1998) Which contrast agent? *Veterinary Practice Nurse* **10**(1), 15–18.

Latham C. (1996) Radiographic film faults and how to avoid them, *Veterinary Practice Nurse* **8**(3), 17–22.

Lee R. (1995) *BSAVA Manual of Small Animal Diagnostic Imaging*, British Small Animal Veterinary Association, Gloucester.

Mendenhall A. and Cantwell H. (1988) *Equine Radiographic Procedures*, Lea and Febiger, Philadelphia.

Middleton D. (1993) Radiographic positioning for the spine and skull, *Veterinary Clinics of North American Small Animal Practice* **23**(2), 253–268.

Perry R. (1993) Principles of conventional radiography and fluoroscopy, *Veterinary Clinics of North American Small Animal Practice* **23**(2), 235–252.

Schramme M. (1999) The lateromedial projection of the foot, *UK Vet* **4**(4), 7–12.

Schramme M. (1998) The dorsopalmar (dorsoproximal–palmarodistal oblique) projection of the distal phalanx, *UK Vet* **3**(6), 7–10.

Smith R. (1999) Tendon scanning. Part 1, *UK Vet* **4**(2), 8–12.

Taffs A. (1997) Senior programmes: where to start, *The Veterinary Nursing Journal* **12**(4), 124–130.

Taylor N. (1999) Indecent exposure, *Veterinary Practice Nurse*, Summer 1999, pp. 10–33.

Torrington A. (2000) Nursing the spinal patient, *Veterinary Practice Nurse*, winter 2000, pp. 19–22.

Tremain H. (2000) Equine dental radiography, *UK Vet* **5**(3), 8–11.

Wilks R. (1987) *Principles of Radiological Physics,* 2nd Edition, Churchill Livingstone.

Wolvekamp W (1994) Basic principles of abdominal radiography, *Vet Q* **16**(Supple 1), 40S–42S.

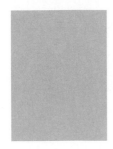

Index